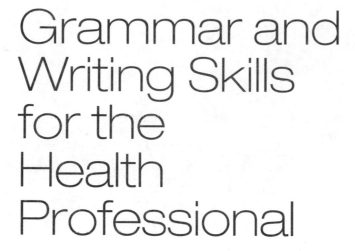

Grammar and Writing Skills for the Health Professional

Dedication

This book is dedicated to those who made it possible:

The Villemaire Family, especially
Norman, Christopher, and Valerie Villemaire, and Robert Oberg

and

The Sisters of St. Joseph of Springfield,
especially Mary Patricia Carr, SSJ

Grammar and Writing Skills for the Health Professional

Lorraine Villemaire, SSJ, MAT, BA

PRESIDENT—CURRICULUM DEVELOPER:

School of Business and Technology

Massachusetts Career Development Institute
Springfield, MA

Doreen Villemaire, MEd., BS, RN, CMA

DEPARTMENT CHAIR:

Medical Assistant Program
Medical Billing and Coding Program

The Salter School
Worcester, MA

PROFESSOR:

Becker College
Worcester, MA

DELMAR
THOMSON LEARNING™

Australia Canada Mexico Singapore Spain United Kingdom United States

DELMAR
THOMSON LEARNING™

Grammar and Writing Skills for the Health Professional

Lorraine Villemaire
Doreen Villemaire

Health Care Publishing Director:
William Brottmiller

Acquisitions Editor:
Maureen Muncaster

Developmental Editor:
Darcy M. Scelsi

Editorial Assistant:
Maria Perretta

Executive Marketing Manager:
Dawn F. Gerrain

Channel Manager:
Tara Carter

Project Editor:
Mary Ellen Cox

Production Editor:
James Zayicek

Art/Design Coordinator:
Jay Purcell

Printed in the United States of America
1 2 3 4 5 XXX 05 04 03 02 01 00

For more information, contact Delmar,
3 Columbia Circle, PO Box 15015,
Albany, NY 12212-0515.

Or find us on the World Wide Web at
http://www.delmar.com

Library of Congress Cataloging-in-Publication Data

Villemaire, Doreen.
Grammar and writing skills for the health professional / Doreen Villemaire, Lorraine Villemaire.
p. cm.
Includes bibliographical references.
ISBN 0-7668-1259-6
1. English language—Grammar—Problems, exercises, etc.
2. English language—Rhetoric—Problems, exercises.
3. Medical writing—Problems, exercises, etc.
I. Villemaire, Lorraine. II. Title.
PE1116.M44 V55 2000
808′.042′02461—dc21

00-060154

NOTICE TO THE READER

Publisher does not warrant or guarantee any of the products described herein or perform any independent analysis in connection with any of the product information contained herein. Publisher does not assume, and expressly disclaims, any obligation to obtain and include information other than that provided to it by the manufacturer.

The reader is expressly warned to consider and adopt all safety precautions that might be indicated by the activities herein and to avoid all potential hazards. By following the instructions contained herein, the reader willingly assumes all risks in connection with such instructions.

The Publisher makes no representation or warranties of any kind, including but not limited to, the warranties of fitness for particular purpose or merchantability, nor are any such representations implied with respect to the material set forth herein, and the publisher takes no responsibility with respect to such material. The publisher shall not be liable for any special, consequential, or exemplary damages resulting, in whole or part, from the readers' use of, or reliance upon, this material.

Contents

Preface

Introducing *Grammar and Writing Skills for the Health Professional* is an exciting endeavor. This book is timely because it is written in an era when health care services are diversifying at an extremely rapid pace. Health care is one of the largest industries in the country today. The constant evolution of health care services and the frequency of litigation have increased the need for meticulous and accurate written communication and documentation. The health care professional, like any other professional, must use correct grammar and writing skills in all types of medical communications.

This book is unique because it addresses the writing concerns of professionals in the medical field. Simplicity is a special feature of the book because it can be easily read and understood. It may be used as a textbook, a manual for staff development, a resource book, or an introductory guide for writing manuscripts, medical reports and documents, grant proposals, and journal articles.

Grammar and Writing Skills for the Health Professional is structured in such a way that grammar, syntax, medical spelling, and other types of medical information are integrated into every chapter. Grammar themes, content, explanations, examples, and exercises are medically oriented and relate to the activities regularly performed in a medical setting. Chapters flow sequentially, beginning with explanations of grammar and applying these skills to the construction of sentences and paragraphs within documentation.

Medical documentation and reports reflect a writing style unique to the medical profession. The writer's choice and arrangement of words are interspersed with medical symbols, abbreviations, and terse phrases. Because of their importance, medical spelling and abbreviations are incorporated into every chapter of the book. Physicians often dictate medical expressions that must be woven into the English language without changing the physician's intent or data. This task requires a good grasp of both the English language and medical language.

The goal for this comprehensive coverage of grammar and writing skills is to simplify and facilitate the writing concerns of health professionals in order that they may provide greater quality health services and care for their patients.

Section One

Grammar Overview

Chapter 1

Nouns

Objectives

Upon completion of this chapter, the student should be able to:

- identify basic types of nouns
- identify nouns by gender, number, and function
- explain the difference between apposition and direct address
- spell various medical terms
- translate various medical abbreviations
- form the plurals of regular nouns and medical nouns

Grammar is a set of rules about words and how they are used in sentences for the purpose of conveying a message. A sentence is a group of words that expresses a complete thought. Words improperly arranged in a sentence cannot be understood, as illustrated in this example:

Classes conference in Carr room Doctor supervisor the arranged.

Rearranged according to the rules of grammar, the words form a logical sentence:

The supervisor, Doctor Carr, arranged classes in the conference room.

The individual words that make up a sentence are called *parts of speech* (see Figure 1-1). They direct the manner in which words are used in sentences. The parts of speech are:

Noun	names a person, place, thing, or idea
Pronoun	substitutes for a noun
Verb	shows action, being, or linking
Adjective	describes a noun or pronoun
Adverb	describes a verb, adjective, or other adverb
Preposition	shows relationship to a noun or pronoun
Conjunction	connects words or groups of words
Article	points out or limits

This section focuses on the different parts of speech and reviews the basic rules of grammar.

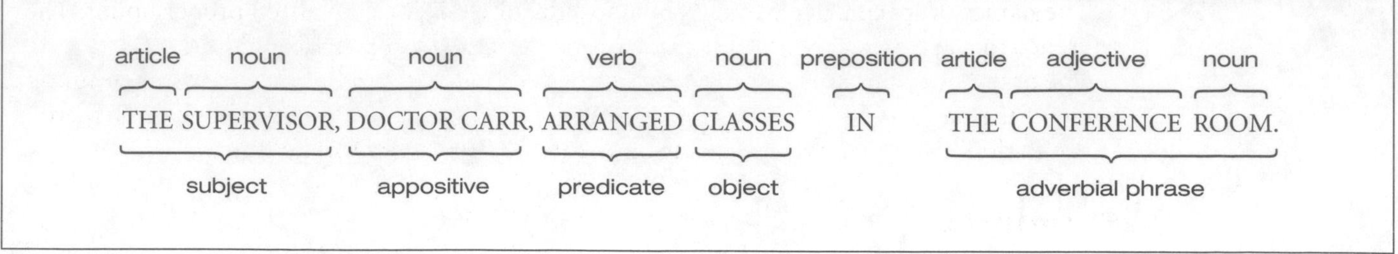

Figure 1-1 Sentence Structure

Types of Nouns

Knowledge of the different types of nouns and how they are used in sentences is essential for accurate medical documentation. Nouns are used more frequently than any other part of speech. Sentences abound with them. Note the number of nouns (in italic) in this sentence:

The *supervisor, Doctor Carr,* arranged *classes* in the conference *room.*

The English language has more nouns than any other part of speech. A noun is a word used to name a person, place, object, (thing, activity), or quality (idea). The types of nouns covered in this chapter are proper, common, collective, concrete, and abstract.

Proper and Common Nouns

Proper and common nouns are easy to understand. A proper noun names a particular person, place, object, or quality. To help remember the definition, think of the words *proper* and *particular* that both begin with the letter *P*. Words like *Main Street, Dr. Villes, Massachusetts, Memorial Hospital, American Association of Medical Assistants (A.A.M.A.), Red Cross,* and *University Hospital* are proper nouns. Proper nouns begin with a capital letter.

Common nouns do not name any specific or particular person, place, object, or quality. They are casual words such as *book, vegetable, hospital, patient, artery, muscle, temperature, admission, bacteria, examination, physician, specimen,* and *bone.* Common nouns do not begin with a capital letter.

Examples

The *physician* [common] worked with the medical *assistant* [common] in the *office* [common].

Dr. Valerie Brown [proper] worked with *Lorry* [proper] in the *Mayo Clinic* [proper].

The *patient* [common] went to the *hospital* [common].

Chris Villes [proper] went to *Mercy Hospital* [proper].

January [proper] is the *month* [common] to review medical *forms* [common].

In the medical field, proper nouns often begin with eponyms. Eponyms are surnames of people used as descriptive adjectives for diseases, instruments, syndromes, procedures, drugs, parts of the human body, and other medical nouns. Words such as Bell's palsy, Babinski's reflex, Foley catheter, and Buck's extension are eponymic terms. The eponym is capitalized, but not the noun following it. It is important to check the spelling of eponyms in a medical dictionary.

The names of specific departments in a hospital or clinic are capitalized proper nouns. The reference to a general department is not a proper noun, and so is not capitalized.

The brand or trade name of a drug is a capitalized proper noun, but the generic or common name of the name is not; for example, aspirin or Bayer aspirin, and meperidine or Demerol. When in doubt about capitalizing, consult the *PDR* (*Physicians Desk Reference*).

Examples

Proper	***Common***
Taber's Cyclopedic Medical Dictionary	chickenpox
German measles	flu
Medical Records Department	operating room
Amoxicillin	penicillin
Tylenol	acetaminophen
Meckel's diverticulum	diverticulitis
Marshall–Marchetti operation	laparotomy

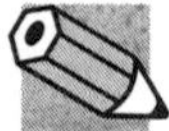

Practice 1-1

Identify the italicized words as proper or common nouns:

1. The largest *artery* in the body is the *aorta.* ________________
2. *Nurses* at the *Mercy Hospital* were not in favor of a *strike.* ________________
3. *Scientists* were watching changes in the *DNA.* ________________
4. *Dr. Sullivan* was an old-fashion *doctor* who went to patients' *homes.* ________________
5. *Dr. Wilson*, on the other hand, sent his *patients* to the emergency *room.* ________________
6. Pulmonary *veins* are the only *veins* in the *body* that carry oxygenated *blood.* ________________
7. *Croup* is the narrowing of the air passage in the *larynx.* ________________
8. The *doctor* said we were going to have another *child.* ________________
9. *Cholesterol* is a lipid found in saturated *fats.* ________________
10. The *patient* had a *Marshall–Marchetti operation.* ________________

Collective Nouns

Collective nouns represent a group of persons, animals, or things. One of the meanings of the word "collective" is a number of people working together. Examples of collective nouns are:

audience	committee	faculty	nation	school
board	company	family	navy	society
choir	crew	group	panel	staff
club	crowd	jury	public	union

Examples

The *staff* of physicians works as a *team.*

The *family* consented to the operation.

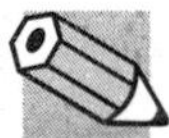

Practice 1-2

Identify the collective nouns in the following sentences.

1. The patient was on the faculty at the medical school. ____________________
2. A group of muscles helps the movement of the mouth. ____________________
3. The association drew up the blueprints for a new wing. ____________________
4. The American Association of Medical Assistants is the group that awards certificates. ____________________
5. The verdict depends on the jury. ____________________
6. Val was a soloist with the choir, chorus, and madrigal singers. ____________________
7. Every nation has its own type of health insurance. ____________________
8. Chris joined the faculty after graduation. ____________________
9. The family is the basic structure of society. ____________________
10. The hospital welcomed the inclusion of a union. ____________________

Concrete Nouns

Concrete nouns are easy to identify because they name things that are touchable, visible, and audible; that is, they are perceived by the senses.

Examples

Bones and *muscles* work together.

Muscles are attached to *bones* by *tendons.*

Massachusetts General Hospital is in *Boston.*

The *New England Journal of Medicine* is an excellent *journal.*

Abstract Nouns

Abstract nouns are more difficult to identify because they name a feeling, quality, or idea. Think of abstract nouns as untouchables. Abstract nouns often have *-ness, -dom, -th, -ance, -cy* and *-ism* for endings. Examples of abstract nouns are:

accuracy	danger	freedom	love	strength
case	emotion	function	memory	theories
concept	energy	grief	method	truth
condition	evidence	honesty	personality	type
courage	foolishness	intelligence	security	

Examples

The *concept* portrayed the *personality* and *honesty* of the individual.

The strength of this *concept* lies in the facts about the musculoskeletal system.

Patience is an admirable *quality* in any medical assistant.

Wordiness is inexcusable in written communication.

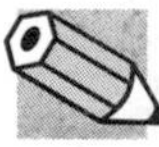

Practice 1-3

State whether the italicized words are collective or abstract:

1. I took the workshop to increase my *confidence.* ____________________

2. The *committee* agreed that *honesty* is the best *policy.* ____________________

3. The Patient's Bill of Rights provides greater *satisfaction* and *care* for the patient. ____________________

4. The medical *staff* is meeting at 10 A.M. ____________________

5. After class, the *group* celebrated its hard work. ____________________

6. *Members* of the A.A.M.A. worked as a *team.* ____________________

7. The *philosophy* of the *group* is *kindness*. ________________

8. I question your *ability* to lead the *board*. ________________

9. Do you have an *opinion* about *religion*? ________________

10. The *evidence* is questionable. ________________

Characteristics and Functions of Nouns

Nouns have three characteristics: gender, number, and case.

Gender

Gender categorizes nouns as masculine, feminine, neuter, or indefinite. Masculine gender words include *men, uncle, boy, rooster, bull,* and *stallion. Mother, girl, woman, queen, hen,* and *daughter* are nouns that belong in the feminine category. Words such as *tree, bicycle, pencil, phone, car, bed, ligament, room, tendons, thermometer, stethoscope,* and *medication* have no male or female references and are called neuter. Neuter nouns are words that can be either masculine or feminine: *president, plumber, parent, doctor, teacher,* and *clerk.*

Why is there a gender for words in the English language? One reason is that writers may wish to vary their text by substituting a pronoun in place of a noun. Gender guides the selection of the correct pronoun. This concept is more fully developed in Chapter 2.

Practice 1-4

State whether the italicized nouns are masculine, feminine, or neuter:

1. The *doctor* won the *award* for the research. ________________

2. Many *men* agree that *women* deserve equal pay. ________________

3. The *winner* of the *prize* was elated. ________________

4. A *tourniquet* was used on the man's *limb*. ________________

5. When visiting the *hospital*, we saw the *nurses* with *signs* at the picket *line*.
____

6. A *biopsy* is the removal of *tissue* from the *body* for examination. ________________

7. The *housekeeper* brushed *cobwebs* from the *closet* in the storage room.
____

8. *Electricians* were called STAT to restore *electricity* for the labs. ________________

9. *Patients* want kindness from their *physicians.* ____________________

10. *Instructors* have a great influence on *students.* ____________________

Number

Number is the form of a noun that indicates whether it is singular (one person or thing) or plural (more than one).

Forming Plurals in General

A few basic rules help to form the plurals of nouns (Figure 1-2). However, like many rules, there are some exceptions. When in doubt about the spelling of any word, always consult a dictionary. If there are two acceptable spellings of plural words given, the first is preferred.

Forming the Plurals of Medical Terms

Many medical terms are derived from Greek and Latin words. Forming the plurals of medical terms is somewhat different than forming the plurals of regular nouns (Figure 1-3). Reviewing the following rules may be helpful when charting, correcting, typing, or corresponding:

1. Most singular nouns are made plural just by adding *s: patient, patients; bone, bones; tendon, tendons; symptom, symptoms; friend, friends; nurse, nurses; write, writes.*
2. To form the plurals of nouns ending in *s, x, ch, sh,* and *z,* add *es: dress, dresses; church, churches; tax, taxes; wish, wishes; quiz, quizzes; process, processes; phalanx, phalanxes; larynx, larynxes.*
3. Singular nouns ending in *y* preceded by a vowel form their plurals by adding *s: attorney, attorneys; boy, boys; x-ray, x-rays; key, keys.*
4. Nouns ending in *y* preceded by a consonant form the plural by changing *y* to *i* and adding *es: policy, policies; copy, copies; allergy, allergies; extremity, extremities; study, studies; dichotomy, dichotomies; deficiency, deficiencies.*
5. Singular nouns ending in *f* and *fe* form the plural in two ways. If the final *f* in the plural form is heard, add *s: belief, beliefs; safe, safes;* and *staff, staffs.* If the final *f* in the plural has a *v* sound, change the *f* to *v* and add *es: life, lives; half, halves; wife, wives; leaf, leaves.*
6. Singular nouns ending in *o* preceded by a vowel form their plurals by adding s: *studio, studios; duo, duos;* and *portfolio, portfolios.* Singular nouns ending in *o* preceded by a consonant form the plural by adding *s or es: echo, echoes; hero, heroes; two, twos; potato, potatoes.* Usage varies, so consult a dictionary when in doubt. Note that there are two acceptable plurals of *zero,* (*zeros, zeroes*) and *no,* (*nos, noes*).

Figure 1-2 Rules for Forming Plurals

1. Change *x* to *c* or *g* and add *es*: *apex, apices; thorax, thoraces; meninx, meninges; appendix, appendices.*
2. Change *is* to *es*: *diagnosis, diagnoses; prognosis, prognoses.*
3. Change *oma* to *omata.*: *stoma, stomata; sarcoma, sarcomata; carcinoma, carcinomata* (but *carcinomas* is also acceptable).
4. Change *a* to *ae*: *sequela, sequelae; vertebra, vertebrae; pleura, pleurae.*
5. Change *um* to *a*: *ovum, ova; bacterium, bacteria; diverticulum, diverticula.*
6. Change *us to i*: *fungus, fungi; streptococcus, streptococci; thrombus, thrombi; bronchus, bronchi.*
7. Change *on* to *a*: *ganglion, ganglia.*
8. Change *en* to *ina*: *lumen, lumina.*

Figure 1-3 Rules for Forming Plurals of Medical Terms

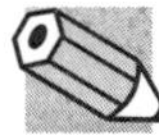

Practice 1-5

Form the plurals of the words in italics.

1. The department ordered *lunch* for the *nurse.* ____________________
2. Protect *child* from electrical shock by covering unused *outlet.* ____________________
3. Maslow arranges human *need* into five *category.* ____________________
4. Many written *form* are required before admission into the hospital. ____________________
5. The *diagnosis* were negative. ____________________
6. The *curriculum* were approved by the *alumnus.* ____________________
7. The *formula* contain many *nutrient.* ____________________
8. Some *patient* in their *seventy* and *eighty* appear more energetic. ____________________
9. Congenital *anomaly* are physical *abnormality* at birth. ____________________
10. There are seven cervical *vertebra.* ____________________

Identify the singular form of these nouns:

1. nuclei   nuclae, nuclons, nucleus   ____________________

2. foci focus, focis, focae ____________

3. strata stratae, strati, stratum ____________

4. emboli emblae, embolum, embolus ____________

5. ova ovae, ovum, ovi ____________

Identify the plural form of these nouns:

1. septum septae, seption, septa ____________

2. fimbria fimbrium, fimbri, fimbriae ____________

3. thorax throaxses, thoraxae, thoraces ____________

4. bronchus bronchae, bronchi, bronchum ____________

5. aponeurosis aponeursum, aponeurosae, aponeuroses ____________

Functions of Nouns

Nouns can be used in different ways in a sentence (see Figure 1-4):

Subject	the person, place, thing, or idea that the sentence is about
Predicate Noun	a word that follows a *being* or *linking* verb and that tells something about the subject
Direct Object	the person, place, thing, or idea that receives the action of the verb

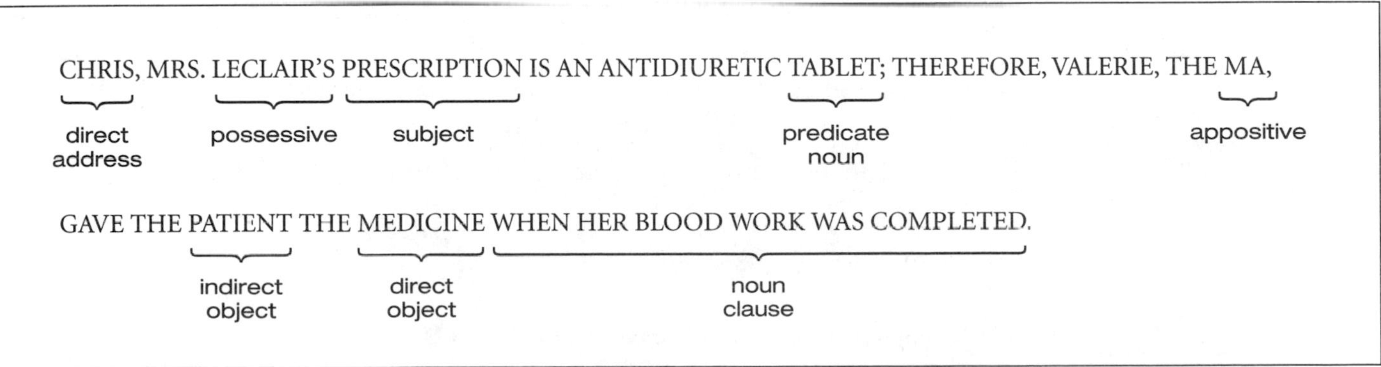
CHRIS, MRS. LECLAIR'S PRESCRIPTION IS AN ANTIDIURETIC TABLET; THEREFORE, VALERIE, THE MA,
direct address
possessive
subject
predicate noun
appositive
GAVE THE PATIENT THE MEDICINE WHEN HER BLOOD WORK WAS COMPLETED.
indirect object
direct object
noun clause

Figure 1-4 Some Uses of Nouns

Indirect Object	a word that answers "to whom?" or "to what?" about the verb
Possessive Noun	a word that indicates possession or ownership by its form
Appositive	a word or group of words following a word to identify or give information about that word
Direct Address	a word or group of words naming or denoting the person or persons spoken to
Noun Phrase or Clause	a group of words used as a noun

The use of a noun in a sentence is described by its case, which basically shows its relationship to other words in the sentence. In English there are three cases: subjective (or nominative), objective, and possessive (or genitive).

Nominative Case: Subject

Nominative case refers to the *subject* (abbreviated S) of a sentence. The subject is always a noun or a group of words that function as a noun. The subject of a sentence is the person, place, thing, or idea about which something is said. It is determined by asking "who?" or "what?" about the verb and can be found anywhere in the sentence.

Examples

The *supervisor* scheduled six nurses. [Who scheduled? The *supervisor* scheduled.]

Students increased their skills with practice. [Who increased? *Students* increased.]

Bones of the skull protect the brain. [What protects? *Bones* protect.]

The *attitude* of our staff makes working in the O.R. enjoyable. [What makes? *Attitude* makes.]

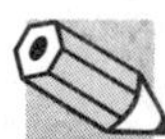

Practice 1-6

Identify the subject in each sentence by placing an S above it:

1. Over the years, my brother remembered his experiences in surgery.
2. The instructor's approach to writing excited the students.
3. The embolus traveled to the lungs.
4. The orthodontist puts braces on the teeth.
5. The symptoms are fever and headache.
6. The ability to proofread is a plus in the doctor's office.
7. The otologist diagnosed otitis media.

8. Your resume must make a good impression in order to get an interview.

9. The radiologist studied the x-ray.

10. The lab technician was our neighbor down the street.

Nominative Case: Predicate Noun

A noun can also function as a subject complement that completes the sense of a verb, or a predicate noun (PN). Sometimes it is referred to as the predicate nominative. It follows immediately after a *being* verb (linking verb): *am, is, are, was, were, have, has, had, be,* or any form of *be* or *been.* It is the same person, place, thing, or idea as the subject.

Examples

Doctors are *specialists.* [*Specialists* is a predicate noun; the word *are* is the being verb.]

Valerie is a good *friend.* [*Friend* is the predicate noun of the subject, *Valerie*; the being verb is *is.*]

Jose Ramos is a medical *assistant.* [*Assistant* is the predicate noun of the subject, *Jose Ramos.*]

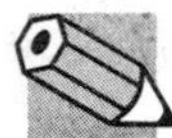

Practice 1-7

Identify the predicate noun in each sentence by placing PN above it:

1. Good articulation is the verbal part of communication.

2. Clothing is a nonverbal message.

3. Communication with patients is an essential skill.

4. Death is a part of the life cycle.

5. Dr. Villes is the doctor on call.

6. Meninges is the term for the protective covering of the brain.

7. This dermatitis is an allergic condition.

8. Access is the database for the program.

9. The patient's response to the illness was denial.

10. The elderly patient is Mrs. Leclair, the CVA in room 513.

Objective Case

Think of the word *object* in connection with the objective case. The direct *object*, the indirect *object*, and the *object* of a preposition constitute the objective case. The direct object and indirect object complete the action of the verb and are found in the predicate.

The direct object (DO) receives the action expressed by the verb. It is found by asking "what?" or "whom?" about the verb.

Examples

The physician dictated a *report.* [Dictated *what*? A *report.*]

Pat discussed *Mary* at the meeting. [Discussed *whom*? *Mary.*]

Can you help *John*? [Help whom? John.]

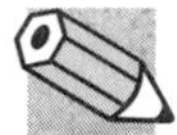

Practice 1-8

Identify the direct object in each sentence by placing DO above it:

1. The neurologist prescribed medication for the condition.
2. The gastroenterologist did the colonoscopy.
3. Patients have a right to information in the medical record.
4. The doctor owns the medical record.
5. The cell contains complex structures.
6. Nurses study biology in college.
7. Court evidence included letters, memos, and tapes.
8. The psychologist treated the patient's depression.
9. The patient suffered allergies in the fall.
10. The oncologist treats cancer patients.

The indirect object (IO) is the noun denoting *to whom, for whom, to what,* or *for what* the action of the verb is being done. It follows the verb and comes before the direct object.

Examples

The patient wrote the *pharmacist* a check. [Wrote *to whom?* The *pharmacist.*]

The entertainer gave the *audience* a real show. [Gave *to whom?* The *audience.*]

Villes Medical Associates pays its *employees* competitive salaries. [Pays to whom? Its *employees.*]

Practice 1-9

Identify the indirect object in each sentence by placing IO above it.

1. The surgeon gave the residents an opportunity to operate.
2. M.A. students showed the instructor the procedure.
3. The nurse gave the patient a johnny.
4. The CNA gave the patient a special delivery letter.
5. Did the lab manager give the technician a raise in pay?
6. The patient mailed the doctor the check.
7. The nurse handed the doctor a scalpel.
8. Matthew told the Medicare class his ideas.
9. The nurse fed the patient some soup.
10. The employer paid his employees an extra week's salary.

The object of a preposition (OP) is the noun that follows a preposition and joins it to other words in the sentence. The preposition along with its object is called a prepositional phrase. The noun that is used as the object of a preposition is never the subject of a sentence.

Some common prepositions are *to, for, on, with, off, in, during, by,* and *over.* Additional prepositions are listed in Chapter 6.

Examples

The doctor wrote a letter *to* the *cardiologist.* [*Cardiologist* is the object of the preposition *to.*]

Arthroscopy is visualization *with* an *endoscope.*

The lady placed the vasodilator medication *under* her *nose.*

Osteomalacia *in children* is called rickets.

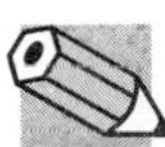

Practice 1-10

Identify the object of the preposition by placing OP above it:

1. The ileum is the distal portion of the small intestines.
2. The medical assistant works in administrative and clinical settings.

3. Ethics is a branch of moral science.

4. CHAMPUS is insurance for military families.

5. A statute of limitations fixes the period of time for legal action.

6. Skills in verbal communication are required of the health-care team.

7. The attitude of the medical assistant should be empathetic.

8. The patient's financial status is in accounts receivable.

Possessive Case

Possessive case indicates possession or ownership. Possessive nouns express something that is part of a person, place, thing, or idea. For example, *patient's medication* shows that the patient is the owner of the medication. *Medication* is the noun that follows the possessive noun, *patient's*. To check the accuracy of the possessive, change the words to *the medication of the patient.*

Use an apostrophe (') to form the possessive. The three rules for forming a possessive noun are listed in Figure 1-5.

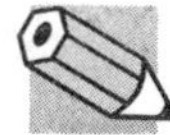

Practice 1-11

Form the possessive of the italicized nouns:

1. Susan enjoyed the *surgeon* demonstrations. ________________

2. *Mr. Archie* office building is for sale. ________________

3. The *doctor* examination revealed no fracture. ________________

4. The *student* grades are passing. ________________

5. Doctors study the *body* anatomy. ________________

6. Everyone voted for *Carol* idea. ________________

7. The *parent* children showed their concern. ________________

8. The *children* dentist is a pedodontist. ________________

9. The dental *technician* surgical scrubs are at the office. ________________

10. The *pharmacy* location is near the atrium of the hospital. ________________

1. To form the possessive of singular nouns, add an apostrophe *s* ('s) to the noun. The word that has the apostrophe is the word that owns something.

   patient's bed [the bed of the patient]

   doctor's white coat [the white coat of the doctor]

2. The possessive of plural nouns ending in *s* is formed by adding only an apostrophe after the *s* (s').

   doctors' dressing room [the dressing rooms of the doctors]

   nurses' scrub gowns [the scrub gowns of the nurses]

   If the plural word does not end in *s*, add an apostrophe and the letter *s* ('s).

   children's diseases [the diseases of children]

3. Irregular nouns not ending in *s* need an apostrophe *s* ('s) to form the possessive.

   The *children's* ward is on the fourth floor.

   The *women's* lounge is down the hall.

4. If two people own an item, only the last name takes the possessive form.

   Lorry and Doreen's book on *Grammar and Writing Skills for the Health Professional* is on the shelf.

   If each person owns the item, both names take the possessive form.

   Dr. Archie's and *Dr. Villes's* stethoscopes are on the treatment table.

5. To form the possessive of singular nouns ending in *s*, add an apostrophe and an *s* ('s).

   Mr. Jones's daughter.

6. To form the possessive of plural nouns ending in *s*, only add an apostrophe (').

   The *Jones'* families.

Figure 1-5 Rules for Forming Possessive Nouns

Appositives and Direct Address

Nouns may also be used as appositives (APP). An appositive is a word or group of words that immediately follows and further identifies another noun. It is usually separated by commas.

Examples

Dr. Villes, *the doctor on call,* performed the ORIF. [The phrase *the doctor on call* identifies and renames the noun, *Dr. Villes.*]

Carr Insurance, *an independent firm,* covered all medical expenses. [The phrase *an independent firm* identifies and renames *Carr Insurance.*]

The noun of direct address (DA) names the listener. The speaker tries to catch the listener's attention by using the person's name. The use of direct address makes messages more direct and personal. Because it interrupts the message, a noun of direct address is separated by commas.

Examples

This equipment, *Miss Archie,* belongs in the treatment room. [The speaker is requesting *Miss Archie* to listen.]

What do you think, *Christopher*?

Sara, please see me after class.

After class, *Sara*, please see me.

Note that commas separate both appositives and nouns of direct address.

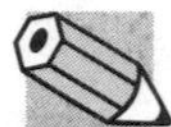

Practice 1-12

Indicate whether the italicized noun or phrase is appositive or direct address by placing APP or DA above it:

1. Tell me, *Doctor*, what is the normal course of treatment for this condition?
2. Do you think, *Dr. Paul,* that the biopsy is necessary?
3. Mr. Newton, *my boss,* will be joining the conference on Wednesday.
4. My husband, *Bob*, developed atrial fibrillation.
5. Schedule an appointment, *Pat*, in six months.
6. Honest, *Abe*, I see no reason why you should run for president.
7. Microsoft Publishers, *a billion-dollar business*, is the leader in the computer arena.
8. Will you faint when you see Paul, *the least likely to succeed*, get all the awards?
9. I've already seen the patient, *Doreen*.
10. The assistant, *Lorry*, set the room up for the next patient.

Nouns Functioning as Phrases or Clauses

A group of two or more words may also function as a noun, either as a noun phrase or a noun clause. Phrases and clauses are nouns when they are used as a subject, direct object, indirect object, or predicate noun.

A noun phrase lacks a subject or a predicate.

To cure disease is the goal of medical research.

The phrase, *To cure disease*, has no subject or predicate. The group of words functions as a noun because it is used as the subject of the entire sentence.

In the following sentence, the phrase is a noun used as a predicate noun after the being verb *is*:

The goal of medical research is *to cure disease.*

A noun clause does contain a subject and a predicate. It can also function as a noun.

The patient didn't understand *why two tests were scheduled.*

The clause, *why two tests were scheduled*, contains a subject (*two tests*) and a predicate (*were scheduled*). The clause in this sentence is a noun that functions as a direct object.

A more in-depth coverage of phrases and clauses is presented in Chapter 7.

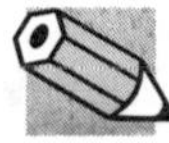

Practice 1-13

Fill in the blanks below with the correct word from the following group:

direct object	appositive	possessive	predicate noun	gender
collective noun	subject noun	abstract noun	proper noun	number

1. Tells what the sentence is about: ________________
2. Names an idea: ________________
3. Refers to a group: ________________
4. Masculine, feminine, neuter: ________________
5. Singular or plural: ________________
6. Follows a linking verb: ________________
7. Receiver of the verb's action: ________________
8. Shows ownership: ________________
9. Renames a noun: ________________
10. Names a particular person, place, or thing: ________________

Identify how the italicized nouns are used in the sentences:

1. *Reports* are dictated by the *physician.*: ________________
2. The *doctor* gave the *nurse* explicit *directions.*: ________________
3. *Nurse,* please administer the *medication* now.: ________________
4. Listen, *Doctor Lee*, the heart is normal.: ________________
5. *Susan* is the best *nurse* on the *floor.*: ________________

Medical Spelling

Become familiar with the spelling of the following words:

allergy, allergies	orthodontist
anesthesiologist	orthopedist
anomaly, anomalies	osteoporosis
appendix, appendices	otitis
bacterium, bacteria	otolaryngologist
biopsy	otologist
bronchus, bronchi	ovum, ova
cardiologist	pathologist
deficiency, deficiencies	pharmacist
dermatologist	pharmacologist
diagnosis, diagnoses	physician
embolus, emboli	process, processes
endocrinologist	psychiatrist
extremity, extremities	psychologist
gastroenterologist	psychosomatic
gynecologist	radiologist
immunologist	stratum, strata
medication	symptoms
neurologist	thorax, thoraces
nucleus, nuclei	thrombus, thrombi
oncologist	urologist
ophthalmologist	vertebra, vertebrae

Nouns Study Summary

Noun	**Names a person, place, thing, or quality.**
Common	Names a *class* of persons, places, objects or qualities: politician, state, author, couple, drug, disease, clinic, company, physician, specimen, virus, therapy, artery, temperature, x-ray.
Proper	Names a *particular* person, place, object, or quality: Republican, Massachusetts, Emily Dickinson, Jack and Jill, Darvon, Hodgkin, Mayo Clinic, Microsoft, Joan Mullins, M.D., Museum of Fine Arts, Basketball

	Hall of Fame, American Medical Association (AMA), American Association of Medical Assistants (AAMA). Proper nouns are capitalized.
Collective	Names a group of persons, animals, or things: government, association, board, public, society, organization, audience, police, nation, flock.
Abstract	Names a quality or idea not perceived by the senses: honesty, goodness, joy, integrity, honor, worth, value, thought, courage, freedom, fear.
Concrete	Names things that are touchable, visible, and audible: pharmacist, therapist, instrument, forceps, alcohol, ointment, medication, hospital.
Gender	**Categorizes nouns as masculine, feminine, neuter, or indefinite.**
Masculine	Represents noun words like male, bull, rooster, Mr.
Feminine	Represents noun words like women, princess, girl.
Neuter	Represents noun words that are neither male nor female: plant, river, desk.
Indefinite	Represents nouns that can be either masculine or feminine: clerk, doctor.
Number	**Categorizes nouns as singular or plural.**
Forming plurals	Add the letter *s* to most nouns: bag, bags; pen, pens; flower, flowers; quota, quotas; and sister-in-law, sisters-in law.
Nouns ending in *s, x, ch, sh, z*	Add *es*: pass, passes; box, boxes; wish, wishes; index, indexes; church, churches; quiz, quizzes.
Nouns ending in *y* preceded by a *vowel*	Add *s* only: boy, boys; key, keys; attorney, attorneys; delay, delays; donkey, donkeys; Saturday, Saturdays.
Nouns ending in *y* preceded by a *consonant*	Change the *y* to *i* and add *es*: city, cities; fly, flies; jalopy, jalopies; dictionary, dictionaries; industry, industries.
Nouns ending in *o* preceded by a *vowel*	Add the letter *s*: studio, studios; shampoo, shampoos; ratio, ratios; stereo, stereos.
Nouns ending in *o* preceded by a *consonant*	Add *s* or *es:* ego, egos; memo, memos; potato, potatoes; hero, heroes; zero, zeros; auto, autos; typo, typos.
Nouns ending in *f* or *fe*	Add the letter *s* if the plural form has an *f* sound: belief, beliefs; proof, proofs; safe, safes; staff, staffs. If the plural form has the *v* sound, change the *f* to *v* and add *es:* life, lives; wife, wives; calf, calves; and loaf, loaves.
Plurals of Medical Nouns	Make the following changes: *x* to *c* or *g* and add *es* : apex, apices; appendix, appendices; thorax, thoraces; phalanx, phalanges. *is* to *es*: diagnosis, diagnoses. *oma* to *omata*: stoma, stomata.

	a to *ae*: sequela, sequelae.
	um to *a*: ovum, ova.
	us to *i*: fungus, fungi.
	on to *a*: ganlion, ganglia.
	en to *ina*: lumen, lumina.
Function	**Categories of usage.**
Nominative	Refers to the subject of the sentence about which something is said.
Subject	"The patient receives excellent care." *Receives excellent care* is what is said about the subject, *patient*.
Predicate Noun	Means the same as the subject but comes right after a being verb. "English is a language." *Language* is the predicate noun that comes after the being verb, *is*.
Objective	Refers to the object of the sentence or preposition.
Direct Object	Directly receives the action of the verb and answers *who* or *what* about the verb. "Students read [*what*?] books." The direct object is *books*.
Indirect Object	Relates indirectly to the verb and answers *to, for whom* and *to, for what* about the verb. "The physician gave [*to whom*?] the patient [*what*?] a prescription." The *patient* is the indirect object.
Object of a Preposition	Follows a preposition and shows its relationship to the rest of the sentence. "The patient came to the office." *Office* is the object of the preposition *to*.
Possessive	Shows ownership or possession.
Singular	Add an apostrophe and *s* to singular nouns: ship's name, Chris's truck, month's allotment, boss's approval.
Plural	Add only an apostrophe to plural nouns ending in *s*: boys' games, heroes' medal.
Irregular	Add an apostrophe and *s*: children's toys, women's blouses
Appositive	Follows a noun and renames it. "The disease, *an inflammation of the spinal cord and brain,* involves the meninges." Note the separation by commas.
Direct Address	Speaks directly to a person and names the listener. "Listen, *Jane*, to the sounds through the stethoscope." Note the separation by commas.
Noun Phrase	Lacks a subject or predicate. "*To alleviate symptoms*, take this medication."
Noun Clause	Contains a subject and a predicate. "*Confidentiality is necessary when health professionals care for patients.*"

Skills Review

Write the noun usage for the italicized word in each sentence: S for subject, DO for direct object, IO for indirect object, OP for object of preposition, APP for appositive, PN for predicate noun., and DA for direct address.

1. The left *knee* was limited in motion due to intrinsic pathology.
2. Hillside Medical Associates pays its *employees* competitive *salaries.*
3. Most *physicians* read several *journals* each week.
4. Joan Arnold, *the supervisor,* is a medical *assistant.*
5. The *AMA* will hold its *election* next month.
6. *Doctors* are *specialists* in their *field.*
7. The patient is a *female* with a *diagnosis* of *gastroenteritis.*
8. The *doctor* gave the *patient* two *prescriptions.*
9. Janet Villes, M.D., *the physician on call,* is easily reached by *phone.*
10. The *nurse* removed the *sutures* from the *incision.*
11. *Visualization* of the *joint* is done with an *endoscope.*
12. To enhance *comfort,* many physicians offer their *patients* better waiting *rooms.*
13. The medical *assistant* transcribed the *report* for the *doctor.*
14. The *patient* is a *man* from the fourth *floor.*
15. *Nurse,* would you please check my *temperature.*
16. *Muscles* can perform a variety of *actions.*
17. Pertinent *findings* about your *patient* are here.
18. *Cramps* are painful *contractions* of *muscles.*
19. The *calcaneus* is the heel *bone.*
20. Seth Wineberg, *the supervisor,* is on *vacation.*

Rewrite these sentences correcting capitals, spellings, possessives, and plurals where necessary:

1. Dr. smith is on call for orthopedic consultation.

 ____

2. Injurie's due to exercise are treated by Orthopedistes.

 ____

3. Bones cannot move without the help of muscles'.

 ____

4. Osteoporosis occurs when bone mass' decreases.

 ____

5. The complexity of the fracture made the operation more difficult.

 ____

6. Bones come in a variety of Sizes and Shapes.

 ____

7. X-Rays in the doctores offices were too old to consult.

 ____

8. the admitting diagnosis is acute intertrochanteric fracture of the Right Hip.

 ____

9. Copys of the report were mailed to the patients physician.

 ____

10. The epiphyses are at the ends of long bone.

 ____

11. Thousands of patients spread bacterium to other workers.

 ____

12. The patients' wishs must be respected.

____

If the noun in italic print is singular, make it plural. If the noun is plural, make it singular.

1. The patient had multiple *diagnosis.* ____________
2. The bacterium responsible for the disease is the *gonococci.* ____________
3. The outer layer of skin has cells that are arranged in *stratum.* ____________
4. In a colostomy, the proximal *stomata* drains the feces. ____________
5. Many *villus* in the small intestines absorb nutrients. ____________
6. Diverticulosis is saclike swellings present in the wall of the colon called *diverticulum.* ____________
7. The blocking of a coronary artery by *thrombi* could lead to an M.I. ____________

Circle the correct plural form of these words. If necessary, check a medical dictionary.

1. antenna — antennas, antenni, antennae
2. extremity — extremities, extremites, extremmities
3. metamorphosis — metamorphos, metamorphos, metamorphoses
4. bacterium — bacteria, bacteri, bacteriac
5. symptom — symptam, symptim, symptoms
6. anomaly — anomilies, anomalys, anomalies
7. diaphysis — diaphysises, diaphyses, diaphysiss
8. vertebra — vertebrum, vertebrae, vertebri
9. process — processes, processos processs
10. phalanx — phalanxes, phalanges, phalanxs

11. diagnosis diagnoss, diagnosiss, diagnosing, diagnoses

12. ganglion ganglionss, ganglia, gangli

Change proper nouns to common nouns and common nouns to proper nouns:

1. The *patient* expects and appreciates courtesy. ____________________
2. Due to an accident, *James* has a greenstick fracture of the right ulna. ____________________
3. The *doctor* praised the *medical assistant* for her efficiency. ____________________
4. The *AMA* is a prestigious group. ____________________
5. Most doctors send their patients to the *Mayo Clinic.* ____________________
6. The *hospital* hired a new *specialist.* ____________________

Translate medical abbreviations using a medical dictionary or appendix.

1. a.c. ____________________
2. AIDS ____________________
3. alt. noc. ____________________
4. AROM ____________________
5. AS ____________________
6. amb ____________________
7. B/S ____________________
8. ASA ____________________
9. B.E. ____________________
10. A&P ____________________

Chapter 2

Pronouns

Objectives

Upon completion of this chapter, the student should be able to:

- identify basic types of pronouns
- identify personal pronouns by gender, number, and function
- use pronouns that agree with their antecedents in number, gender, and person
- spell various medical terms
- translate various medical abbreviations

Once upon a time there was a medical office unit with four medical assistants named *Everybody*, *Somebody*, *Anybody*, and *Nobody*. There was an important job to be done, and *Everybody* was sure that *Somebody* would do it. *Anybody* could have done it, but *Nobody* did it. *Somebody* got angry with this because it was *Everybody*'s job. *Everybody* thought *Anybody* could do it, but *Nobody* realized that *Everybody* wouldn't do it. It ended up that *Everybody* blamed *Somebody* when *Nobody* did what *Anybody* could have done. (Author unknown)

Welcome to the world of pronouns. A pronoun is a word that replaces or substitutes for a noun; for example:

> *Leah* borrowed *books* from the library. *She* returned *them* yesterday.

Note that the pronouns *she* and *them* take the place of the nouns *Leah* and *books*.

Because of the close relationship between nouns and pronouns, there are a lot of similarities in how both are used in sentences. Therefore, anyone with a good understanding of nouns will have no difficulty with pronouns.

Types of Pronouns

The different types of pronouns are personal, reflexive, relative, indefinite, interrogative, and demonstrative. The meaning of each pronoun is contained within its name, which makes them easier to understand:

- Personal pronouns refer to persons (and things).
- Reflexive pronouns throw back or reflect.
- Relative pronouns relate to other words.
- Indefinite pronouns refer to the unknown.
- Interrogative pronouns ask questions.
- Demonstrative pronouns point out or demonstrate.

Personal Pronouns

Personal pronouns refer to specific people and things. They are used more frequently than any other pronoun. Personal pronouns have three characteristics: gender, number, and person. They are also distinguished by case, being either nominative, objective, or possessive. Choosing which personal pronoun to use depends on how it is used in a sentence.

Personal Pronouns

I, you, he, she, it, we, you, they
me, you, it, us, you, their, theirs
my, mine, your, yours, his, her, hers, its, our, ours, your, yours, and them

Gender

Like nouns, pronouns are characterized by gender: masculine, feminine, neuter, and indefinite. Masculine pronouns are *he, his, him.* Feminine pronouns are *she, her, hers.* Indefinite pronouns represent unknown persons or things, such as *all, anything, someone.* The word *it* is an example of a neuter pronoun.

Examples

He is very protective of *his* property. [masculine]

Anyone can be successful. [indefinite]

It belongs to the person who finds *it*, I believe. [neuter]

She was all ears after *she* learned about *her* grades. [feminine]

Number and Person

Number is about whether a pronoun refers to one person or thing (singular) or more than one (plural). Person denotes whether one is speaking (first person), spoken to (second person), or spoken about (third person). Table 2-1 shows pronoun forms categorized by person and number.

Table 2-1 Number and Person of Pronouns

		Number	
Person	**Meaning**	**Singular**	**Plural**
First	Speaker	I, me, my, mine	we, us, our, ours
Second	Individual addressed	you, your, yours	you, your, yours
Third	Person or thing spoken about	he, she, it, his, her, hers, its	they, their, theirs, them

Examples

I am always right. [first person singular]

We are at the medical conference. [first person plural]

My schedule is very busy. [first person singular]

You should check the treatment room for antiseptics. [second person singular or plural]

You make *your* own way. [second person singular or plural]

He said the matter could be settled now. [third person singular]

They should have signed the medical consent form. [third person plural]

The anatomy books belong to *them*. [third person plural]

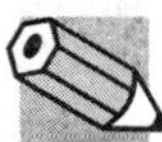

Practice 2-1

Use Table 2-1 to identify the italicized pronouns in the following sentences as first, second, or third person and singular or plural:

1. The exam took a long time but *it* was simple. ________________
2. The instructor showed the procedure to *her* class. ________________
3. Are they *your* new patients? ________________
4. Are you talking to *me?* ________________
5. The time is *ours* for the taking. ________________
6. *You* should know more about *them* than I do. ________________
7. The medical history given to *us* was complete. ________________
8. Betsy is welcomed if *she* follows the policy. ________________
9. Mary was late for *her* class. ________________
10. *They* found a kidney stone in the strainer. ________________

The choice of pronouns depends on how they function in a sentence, and that is where case comes in.

Nominative Case

The subject pronoun—*I, you, he, she, it, we,* and *they*—is the person or thing talked about in a sentence.

Examples

He tripped on the stairs.

They work at the Medical Center.

She is the Chief Resident.

I felt confident I could do the job.

Although the bronchoscopy was simple, *it* took a long time to do.

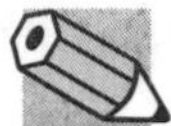

Practice 2-2

Choose the correct pronoun from within the parentheses:

1. (Me, I) visited my best friend who is in the hospital.

2. Mr. Jones, (you, your) have no idea how much work is involved in preparing the patient.

3. (He, Him) and (I, me) were chosen for the positions.

4. (She, Her) answered the office telephone immediately.

5. (It, Its) doesn't make any difference what the EKG reads.

6. Jill, Debbie, and (I, me) joined the AAMA.

7. (They, Them) arrived as the patient returned from the recovery room.

8. (We, Us) were turned away at the laboratory.

9. As transcriptionists, (we, us) stand behind our work.

10. (You, Your) and (she, her) make a good team.

Predicate pronouns are the same as subject pronouns: *I, you, he, she, it, we, they*. They are found after a being verb: *am, is, are, was, were, have, has, had, be,* or *been.*

Examples

The visitor must have been *she*.

Is *she* the owner?

Is it *I*?

It is *she* who pays the bill.

Was it *he* who called?

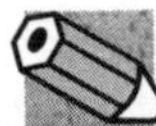

Practice 2-3

Choose the correct predicate pronoun from within the parentheses:

1. The student is (her, she).
2. Is (she, her) the office manager?
3. The medical personnel on the case were (us, we).
4. It was (me, I) who administered cardiopulmonary resuscitation.
5. The dental hygienists are (they, them).
6. The resident who did the physical exam on the patients was (he, him)
7. Is it (she, her) that has the diagnosis of hypertension?
8. The cholecystectomy patient is (it, she).
9. This is (her, she) with the antiseptic solution.
10. Born in a foreign country, (them, they) felt fearful and uneasy in the hospital.

Objective Case

A pronoun that receives the action of the verb either directly or indirectly is an object pronoun.

The direct object pronoun—*me, you, him, her, it, us, you them*—receives the action of the sentence.

Examples

The hemorrhoids gave *her* pain.

The patient paid *them* in cash.

Laurie helped *me* with the amniocentesis.

The indirect object pronoun, like the noun, receives the indirect action of the verb.

The indirect object pronouns are the same as the object pronouns: *me, you, him, her, it, us, you, them.*

Examples

Dr. Rodriguez gave *you* some medication.

The change in surgical procedures saved *them* time.

The AMA loaned *us* medical literature.

Evelyn sent *me* the x-ray report.

Pronouns that follow a preposition are also objective: *me, you, him, her, it, us, you,* and *them.*

Examples

I gave the sphygmomanometer to *them.*

Jane spoke to *her* several times on the phone.

It was a good thing for *them* to do.

English is taught to *her* and *me.*

Possessive Case

The possessive case shows ownership or possession. The possessive pronouns are *my, mine, our, ours, his, her, hers, their, theirs, its,* and *yours.*

Examples

The patient refused to eat *his* food.

The blue lab coat is *mine.*

The urinalysis is *hers.*

Table 2-2 provides a review of the personal pronouns categorized by case.

Table 2-2 Cases of Personal Pronouns

Nominative Case	Objective Case	Possessive Case
Subject and predicate pronouns: I, you, he, she, it, we, they	Direct and indirect object or object of a preposition: me, you, him, her, it, us, you, them	Possessive pronouns: my, mine, you, yours, his, her, hers, its, our, ours, their, theirs

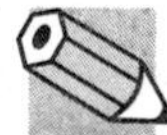

Practice 2-4

Select the correct pronoun from within the parentheses. State how it is used in each sentence: subject, predicate, direct object, indirect object, object of a preposition, or possessive.

1. (He, Me) had no idea about the aneurysm. ____________________

2. The medical assistant helped (me, I) with the medical record. ____________________

3. I carried a stethoscope with (me, I). ____________________

4. This is (her, she) giving the antibiotics. ____________________

5. (Them, They) should get the electrocardiogram from (he, him) ____________________

6. Luke and (me, I) are physician-employers. ____________________

7. The CPT coding books are (mine, me). ____________________

8. (Her, Hers) bronchoscopy showed carcinoma of the lungs. ____________________

9. The medical assistant showed (he, him) the x-ray. ____________________

10. Is (she, her) doing the urinalysis? ____________________

Reflexive Pronouns

Reflexive pronouns reflect back to the person. To form them, add *self* or *selves* to the personal pronoun. Depending on how it is used in the sentence, a reflexive pronoun can be a direct object, indirect object, object of a preposition, or a predicate pronoun.

Reflexive Pronouns
myself, himself, herself, itself, yourself, themselves, ourselves

Examples

She buys *herself* a stethoscope. [indirect object]

He gives *himself* insulin injections every day. [indirect object]

I am *myself* only when I feel good. [predicate pronoun after the being verb *am*]

They smiled at *themselves* when the procedure was over. [object of a preposition]

Practice 2-5

Provide the correct reflexive pronoun:

1. I enjoyed ____________________ at the conference on Medical Coding and Billing.

2. Doreen and Val enjoyed ____________________ too.

3. Do you appreciate ____________________ enough to rest once in a while?

4. Lorry volunteered the information ____________________.

5. As for ____________________, I prefer to work in the clinical setting.

6. We pat ________________ on the back when we balance the accounts.

7. Dr. Archie gave ________________ an hour to complete the amniocentesis.

8. Giving to others is a reward in ________________.

9. To complete the manuscript, we will do it ________________.

10. John canceled the appointments ________________.

Relative Pronouns

Relative pronouns relate one part of a sentence to a word in another part of the sentence.

Relative Pronouns
who, which, that

A relative pronoun helps to join a relative clause to the rest of the sentence. The most important relative pronouns are *who, which,* and *that.*

Who refers to people.

Examples

The patient *who* needs the antiemetic is in room 430.

Who is the relative pronoun.

Who is the relative pronoun that refers to the patient.

The physician *who* ordered the procedure is on rounds.

Which refers to things. *Which* is used when the clause that it introduces is not essential to the meaning of the sentence.

Examples

The medical record, *which* is confidential, shows the diagnosis.

The crash cart, *which* is used for emergencies, needs to be restocked.

That refers to people or things. *That* is used when the clause that it introduces is essential to the meaning of the sentence.

Examples

The type *that* is needed for this wound is a figure eight bandage.

The doctor wrote the letter *that* has the information.

Practice 2-6

Select the correct pronoun:

1. The patient has Dr. Villes, (who, that) is scheduled to go on vacation tomorrow.
2. Diagnostic tests, (which, who) are used for cardiopathy, should be read by a cardiologist.
3. Disbursements, (which, who) are made in the office, are recorded in the check register.
4. This is the telemetry (which, that) records the heart rate.
5. The electrocardiograph, (which, who) we used yesterday, is not working.
6. Progress notes (who, that) are documented in various styles, are legal documents.
7. The patient had cryotherapy (who, that) included cold compresses.
8. The MA (which, who) took the History and Physical is working in the clinic.
9. This is the patient (which, who) needs the lab test.
10. This is the centrifuge (who, that) Chris prefers to use.

Indefinite Pronouns

Indefinite pronouns refer to persons or things in general. Most indefinite pronouns are singular and require a singular verb.

Indefinite Pronouns

all, another, any, anybody, anyone, anything, both, each, each one, either, everybody, everyone, everything, few, many, most, much, neither, nobody, none, no one, nothing, one, other, several, some, somebody, someone, something, such

Examples

Each of the employees wants [singular verb] *her* surgical scrubs ordered through the catalog.

Anyone who gives [singular verb] to charity is twice blessed.

Neither person knows [singular verb] the correct answer.

Every pharmaceutical company has *its* own sales person.

Everyone will send *his/her* consultation to the medical team by Friday.

Plural indefinite pronouns, such as *both, many, few,* and *several,* are used with the plural possessive pronoun, *their.*

Examples

Many on the medical staff expressed *their* concerns about the care given to patients.

Several voiced *their* anger.

All staff members are to report to *their* stations.

Most parents want the best for *their* children.

The indefinite pronouns *all, some, any,* and *none* are either singular or plural depending on how they are used in a sentence.

Examples

None of the equipment is [singular verb] modern.

All the students knew *their* abbreviations by heart.

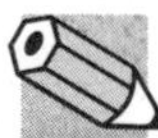

Practice 2-7

Write S if the pronoun is singular and P if the pronoun is plural.

1. Either of the girls can perform her procedure. ____________________

2. Each of the books was returned to its proper place. ____________________

3. Many of the assistants brought their dictation equipment. ____________________

4. Both raised their quality standards. ____________________

5. Few of the pharmacies wanted their prices to increase. ____________________

6. Each thought about his/her place in history. ____________________

7. All have their own respiratory therapists. ____________________

8. Everyone expects his/her resume to be finished before graduation. ____________________

9. No one offered to do his job in the outpatient department. ____________________

10. None of these people want his/her health premiums to increase. ____________________

Interrogative Pronouns

Interrogative pronouns are used simply to ask questions. They are *who, whom, whose, which,* and *what.* Note that some of these pronouns are also relative.

Interrogative Pronouns
who, whose, whom, which, what

Examples

Who ordered this type of medication?

What caused the fever?

Demonstrative Pronouns

The easiest pronouns to learn are the demonstrative pronouns: *this, that, these,* and *those.* They point out. The singular pronouns *this* and *that* point out people or things that are near in space or time. *These* and *those* are plural pronouns referring to people or things that are farther away in space or time.

Demonstrative Pronouns
this, that, these, those

When writing, place a noun right after the demonstrative pronoun to make the sentence clearer.

Examples

This is the first restaurant on the street. [The demonstrative pronoun *this* points out the *restaurant.*]

These need sterilizing.

That was a good decision.

Those are rare tumors.

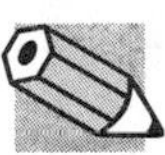

Practice 2-8

Identify the pronouns as demonstrative or interrogative:

1. This needs to be filed in medical records. ____________________

2. Who was responsible for the travel itinerary? ____________________

3. These are the suture scissors. ___________________

4. Which is your health insurance plan? ___________________

5. Whom do you know is providing that coverage? ___________________

6. Those are found with the retractors. ___________________

7. Who read the EKG? ___________________

8. What are you reading? ___________________

9. What is the proper hand washing technique? ___________________

10. To whom do you wish to speak? ___________________

Practice 2-9

Identify each pronoun as personal, reflexive, relative, indefinite, interrogative, or demonstrative:

1. The medical report was given to me to transcribe. ___________________

2. Who would think the illness was a malignancy? ___________________

3. We have to sterilize the instruments ourselves. ___________________

4. These are the ones needed at the Grand Rounds. ___________________

5. Nobody offered to help us. ___________________

6. None of the charts is in its place. ___________________

7. The doctor examined his patient. ___________________

8. The students gave their instructor full attention. ___________________

9. I didn't know the etiology of the disease. ___________________

10. They were the first people to apply for the position. ___________________

Pronoun-Antecedent Agreement

The noun that a pronoun replaces is called its antecedent. All pronouns have noun antecedents. The antecedent usually appears before the noun.

Bill applied an *antiseptic*. He applied *it*.[*Bill* is the antecedent for the pronoun *he* and *antiseptic* is the antecedent for the pronoun *it*.]

Pronouns may also be antecedents of other pronouns.

He took *his* antibiotics. [*He* is the antecedent of *his*.]

Pronouns must agree with their noun antecedents in three ways: number, gender, and person.

Number

Use a singular pronoun to refer to a singular noun.

Alice wants *her* report finished today. [*Alice* and *her* are singular.]

Use plural pronouns to refer to plural nouns.

The *Smiths* are giving a party at *their* home. [*Smiths* and *their* are plural.]

When antecedents are joined by *or* or *nor*, the pronoun agrees with the antecedent nearest to the pronoun.

Examples

Neither Jim nor the *assistants* want *their* positions taken away. [The word *assistants* is closer and plural, so the plural pronoun *their* is used.]

Either Mary or *Ellen* wants to do *her* share.

Use a plural pronoun when two antecedents are joined by the word *and*.

Harry and I think *we* need a raise in pay.

Gender

Use masculine, feminine, or neuter pronouns depending on the gender of their antecedents.

Examples

The *man* brought *his* antibiotics to work. [*Man* and *his* are masculine.]

Mary increased *her* skills with practice. [*Mary* and *her* are feminine.]

The *tracing* is irregular, *it* shows artifacts. [*Tracing* and *it* are neuter.]

When in doubt about the gender, two options are possible:

1. Use *his/her*: One of the students bought *his or her* book.
2. Make the noun plural and use the plural pronoun: *Students* bought *their* books.

Person

Recall that the first person is the speaker, the second person is the individual addressed, and the third person is the person or thing spoken about. In the sentence, "*Mary* likes *her* aerosols kept in the closet," *Mary* is the first person singular noun, so a first person singular pronoun must be used: *her*. In "The *girls* left *their* books at the library," *girls* is third person plural noun and *their* is a third person plural pronoun. Finally, consider the following sentences:

Bill changed the *catheters*. *He* changed *them*.

Bill is first person singular and *he* is first person singular. The antecedent *catheters* is third person plural and its pronoun, *them*, is third person plural.

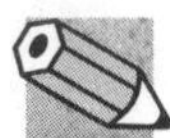

Practice 2-10

Identify the antecedent of the pronoun in each sentence:

1. You must wait *your* turn. ________________
2. Alex and Rene like *their* new office. ________________
3. David improved *his* grades. ________________
4. I completed *my* term paper. ________________
5. The doctor wrote *his* cerebrovascular article. ________________
6. The patient corrected *his* insulin injection. ________________
7. Val and I practiced *our* medical terminology. ________________
8. Pat wondered if *she* qualified. ________________
9. The doctor felt the patient's face. *It* was hot. ________________
10. Medical personnel should know *their* CPR technique. ________________

Select the correct pronoun from within the parentheses:

1. The instructors planned (her/his, their) classes.
2. I stand by (my, mine) principles.
3. Neither Joan nor Pat reached (their, his/her) goal.
4. Kathy and Bill calibrated (their, his/her) instruments.
5. Nobody lost (his/her, their) place.
6. Bill and (she, her) went to (her, their) class on cardiopulmonary resuscitation.
7. When a patient has a cerebrovascular accident, (they, she/he) may become hemiplegic.
8. Some people develop hypertension as (they, his/her) get older.

9. They plan to explain (their, them) reasons for diagnosing pancreatitis.

10. Can you and the committee give us (their, them) decision?

Commonly Confused: The Use of Its and It's

It — Used only to refer to a specific noun: "When the *code alarm* rings, *it* can be heard a mile away."

Its — The possessive pronoun: "The *stethoscope* is missing *its* diaphragm."

It's — The contraction for "it is." The apostrophe is the sign that the word is used as a contraction: "*it's* a normal EKG" means "*it is* a normal EKG."

One way to check the correct usage of "it's" is to say *it is* instead when reading the sentence. For example, in "The computer printed (it's, its) hardcopy," using *it's* would make it read: "The computer printed *it is* hardcopy." That is not correct. The possessive, *its*, shows that the computer owns the hardcopy, and that is the correct form of the pronoun to use.

Medical Spelling

Become familiar with the spelling of the following words:

aerosols	conjunctiva
amniocentesis	electrocardiogram
antibiotics	esophagus
aneurysm	etiology
antiemetic	fallopian tube
antiseptic	fontanel
auscultation	gallbladder
bronchoscopy	glaucoma
cardiopulmonary resuscitation (CPR)	hemiplegic
cataract	hemorrhoids
catheter	hypertension
cerebrovascular	hypotension
cholecystectomy	insulin
cirrhosis	meninges
coagulation	mesentery

occlusion	prostatitis
palpitations	quadriplegia
pancreas	sphygmomanometer
pancreatitis	stethoscope
paraplegia	urinalysis

Pronoun Study Summary

Pronoun	**A word that replaces or substitutes for a noun.**
Personal	Refers to persons. *Singular*: I, me, my, mine, you, your, yours, he, she, it, his, hers, its. *Plural*: we, us, our, ours, you, your, yours, they, their, theirs, them
Reflexive	Reflects, throws back: myself, himself, herself, itself, yourself, themselves, ourselves.
Relative	Relates to other words: who, whose, whom, which, what, that, whomever, whichever, whatever
Indefinite	Refers to persons or things in general: all, another, any, anybody, anyone, anything, both, each, each one, either, everybody, everyone, everything, few, many, most, much, neither, nobody, none, no one, nothing, one, other, several, some, somebody, someone, something, such
Interrogative	Asks questions: who, whose, whom, which, what
Demonstrative	Points out, demonstrates: this, that, these, those.

Usage Forms

	Subjective (subject)	Objective (object)	Possessive with Noun	Possessive without Noun	Reflexive (same person or thing as subject)
Singular					
First person	I	me	my	mine	myself
Second person	you	you	your	yours	yourself
Third person	he, she, it	him, her, it	his, her, its	his, her, its	himself herself itself
Plural					
First person	we	us	our	ours	ourselves
Second person	you	you	your	yours	yourself
Third person	they	them	their	theirs	themselves

Antecedent The noun that is replaced by a pronoun. Pronouns must agree with their noun antecedents in three ways: number, gender, and person.

Number

Singular: *Bill* took the EKGs. *He* took five.

Plural: The *doctors* gave *their* off duty time to volunteer.

Gender

Masculine singular: *Jonathan* liked *his* care.

Feminine plural: *Medical assistants* wear *their* hair at a certain length.

Person

1st (speaker): *Norma* is my name. *I* am named after my father Norman.

2nd (spoken to): *Pat,* are you sure? Do *you* mean what you say?

3rd (spoken about): *Norman and Leonard* know how to scrub. *They* understand surgical technique.

Antecedents joined by *and* need a plural pronoun: *Tom and Mary* are friends. *They* study together.

For antecedents joined by *or* or *nor*, the pronoun agrees with the nearest antecedent: Either the doctor or the *nurses* left *their* charts here.

Skills Review

Circle the correct pronoun from within the parentheses:

1. Each procedure has (its, their) own requirements.
2. Lorry and (she, her) were getting the patient ready for the cholecystectomy.
3. (Who, Whom) did the cross-reference on these files?
4. The doctor appointed (he, him) to the Quality Assurance Program.
5. Someone called with a medical office emergency. I did schedule (him, them) STAT.
6. Luke formatted the disks with Chris and (I, me).
7. It was (she, her) who established the matrix on the appointment schedule.
8. One of the patients developed (his, their) symptoms over two years.
9. Norm and (I, me) are leaving for the conference in the morning.
10. (Who, Whom) shall we hire to do the insurance claims?
11. The PT (coagulation test) was done by (we, us).
12. (She, Her) has an abnormally high concentration of sugar in the blood, indicating hyperglycemia.

13. It could have been (they, them) who gave prior authorization.
14. Because all did (his, their) share, the medical staff were able to leave early.
15. Show Carol and (we, us) your new stethoscope.
16. (I, me) used a fine brush to clean the electrodes.
17. (Who, Whom) can I credit for this organized brochure?
18. I noticed that someone left (his, their) book in the classroom.
19. Patient confidentiality is extremely important to (we, us).
20. With (who, whom) are you going?
21. The ward clerk was quite helpful to (we, us).
22. One of the medical assistants lost (his, their) stethoscope.
23. (Who, Whom) was promoted to Chief Resident of Surgery?
24. The instruments were put in a sanitizing solution while Norman and (I , me) washed our hands.

Circle the indefinite pronoun and above it write S if singular or P if plural:

1. Everyone suffering from orthopnea must sit up to breathe.
2. Good students study hard and most will succeed.
3. Both of them are good medical assistants.
4. Not one of the orthopedic patients has traction.
5. All must report to the office immediately.
6. Many of our students realize that their oral communication skills are vital to their success.
7. Mrs. Gallway believes that few of our administrative assistants are familiar with that procedure.
8. Although Dr. Villes wanted Brian and Tom, neither were available.

9. The tumors were not visible, but he found several when he conducted the examination.

10. None of the symptoms indicated an emergency.

Circle the correctly spelled word in each line:

1. coagulation	caogulation	coaguletion	coaggulation
2. antimetic	cataract	mininges	cirhosis
3. prostetitis	prostattitis	prostatetis	prostatitis
4. esofagus	oclusion	aerosols	anteseptic
5. hemorhoids	hemmorrhoids	hemorrhaids	hemorrhoids
6. insulin	misentery	cateter	anurysm
7. urenalysis	hypotension	cholecystectamy	meningis
8. eteology	cerebrovescular	broncuscopy	etiology
9. antibiotics	arosols	antibiautics	glowcoma
10. electrokardiogram	electrocardigram	electrocardiogram	eletrocardiogram

Translate medical abbreviations using a medical dictionary or appendix.

1. b.i.d. ____________________

2. BUN ____________________

3. BPH ____________________

4. CABG ____________________

5. Bx ____________________

6. CBC ____________________

7. C/O ____________________

8. COPD ____________________

9. C&S ____________________

10. C/C ____________________

Chapter 3

Verbs

Objectives

Upon completion of this chapter, the student should be able to:

- identify verb types
- define the difference between transitive and intransitive verbs
- use verbs that agree with the subject in number and person
- distinguish between active and passive voices
- form the principal parts of regular and irregular verbs
- use the simple past, present and future tenses correctly
- understand how the mood of verbs affects the action of a sentence
- spell various medical terms
- translate various medical abbreviations

Types of Verbs

Verbs are *the* essential components of sentences. They denote action or being. Verbs are a challenge to master because they have a variety of forms that perform many functions.

Action Verbs

Action verbs are words that express activity, both physical and mental.

Examples

Blood *circulates* through the heart, arteries, and veins.

Ask for an appointment.

The patient *complains* of extreme thirst.

The doctor *performed* the operation.

He *proved* his point.

The doctor *evaluates* the physical and mental condition of the patient.

Being Verbs

Verbs can also express a state of being. Being verbs were introduced in Chapter 2 in connection with predicate pronouns. Any form of the verb *to be* that stands alone is a being verb: *am, is, are, was, were, have, has, had,* or any form of *be* or *been.*

Examples

I *am* the nurse in charge.

Bob *is* the patient in question.

We *were* watching for obvious symptoms.

I *have* instructions for such emergencies.

Being verbs may be used as the only verb in a sentence or they may be combined with another verb. When a being verb is used with another verb, it can be a linking verb, a helping verb, an auxiliary verb, or a verb phrase.

Examples

I *was* at the hospital.	I *was helping* the nurse.
Phil *did* his procedures.	Philip *did mention* that fact.
The exam *was* thorough.	They *had found* the exam very thorough.

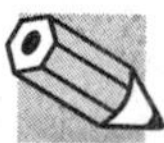

Practice 3-1

Identify the verb in each sentence:

1. Antibiotics are expensive. ____________________
2. Patricia wore a lab coat to dinner. ____________________
3. Cataracts are common in the elderly. ____________________
4. Hands washed frequently prevent the transmission of disease. ____________________
5. Carol irrigates the wound. ____________________
6. The patient signed the consent form. ____________________
7. The doctor, who taught anatomy, retired from teaching. ____________________
8. Palpation is one of the five Ps. ____________________
9. Tetracycline is a broad-spectrum antibiotic. ____________________
10. The pain radiates to her shoulder. ____________________

Main Verbs and Helping Verbs

A single verbs in a sentence is called the main verb:

Janet *disclosed* the information. The dentist *cleaned* the teeth.

Sometimes the main verb is accompanied by one or more helping verbs. The most common helping verbs are *is, are, was, were, am, been, shall, will, would, did, must, can, could, may, might, ought, have, had, has, do,* and *should.* The combination of a helping verb and a main verb is referred to as a verb phrase. In a verb phrase, the last verb is always the main verb.

Examples

The patient *can eat* solid foods. [*Can* is the helping verb and *eat* is the main verb.]

The intern *had studied* all night. [*Had* is the helping verb and *studied* is the main verb.]

The committee *will appoint* the secretary. [The verb phrase is *will appoint.*]

Operations *were delayed* for one hour. [The verb phrase is *were delayed.*]

Verbs may be separated by other words that are not part of the verb phrase.

Examples

Mark *has* never *liked* working in the laboratory.

Can Dr. Villmarie *operate* next Thursday?

Helping verbs may also stand alone as the main verb:

May Tom leave the room? Yes, he *can.*

Linking Verbs

A linking verb connects a complement. A complement is a word or phrase that completes the meaning of a linking verb. Common linking verbs are *is, are, was, were, have, has, had,* and any form of *be* or *been.* Other linking verbs are *feel, grow, seem, stay, taste, appear,* and *become.* The complement may be a predicate noun, pronoun, or adjective (describer).

Examples

Mary *is* my *assistant.* [*Is* is the linking verb, *assistant* is the complement (predicate noun).]

John *is* the *supervisor.* [*Is* is the linking verb, *supervisor* is the complement (noun).]

The employees *were they.* [*Were* is the linking verb, *they* is the complement (pronoun).]

The ideas *are excellent.* [*Are* is the linking verb, *excellent* is the complement (adjective).]

Mr. Williams *appeared angry.* [*Appeared* is the linking verb, *angry* is the complement (adjective).]

Sometimes linking verbs may be separated by other words in the sentence.

Examples

Tim *has* never *administered* medications.

John *has* already *stabilized* the patient's blood pressure.

Practice 3-2

Identify the verb or verb phrases in each sentence:

1. John tolerates the procedure well. ____________________
2. The nail punctured the skin. ____________________
3. I should have been informed. ____________________
4. We have read the article in the journal. ____________________
5. Can Rose operate the computer? ____________________
6. A patient has the right to privacy. ____________________
7. Has the B.P. been stabilized? ____________________
8. Fluid accumulated in the lungs. ____________________
9. Caffeine stimulates the nervous system. ____________________
10. His condition deteriorated rapidly. ____________________

Transitive and Intransitive Verbs

A transitive verb shows action and needs a direct object to complete its meaning.

Examples

The patient ate solid *food.* [*Food* is the *direct object,* so the verb is transitive.]

The anesthesiologist intubated the *patient.*

The surgeon sutured the *laceration.*

The surgical team changed scrub *clothes.*

Verbs that do not have a direct object are called intransitive verbs. These verbs have no object to receive the action.

Examples

The patient ate poorly. [There is no direct object so the verb is intransitive.]

The surgeon sutured.

Cancer radiates quickly from the lymph nodes.

The students studied for three hours.

The surgical team changed.

Practice 3-3

Identify the verbs and indicate whether they are transitive or intransitive:

1. The tumor damaged many muscles. ________________
2. The temperature recurred. ________________
3. The physician placed ointment on the wound. ________________
4. The doctor introduced the scope. ________________
5. The music relaxed the surgical team in the OR. ________________
6. The IV punctured the skin. ________________
7. The trachea bifurcates into the right and left bronchi. ________________
8. The patients sat in wheelchairs along the hall. ________________
9. The test reveals normal blood cholesterol. ________________
10. The instruments were sterilized. ________________

Verbals

Verbs can also function as nouns, adjectives, or adverbs. These forms are called verbals. Gerunds and infinitives are verbals. A gerund is formed by adding *ing* to the verb. An infinitive is formed by placing *to* in front of the verb.

Examples

Operating is the surgeon's occupation. (Gerund)

To work with you is a pleasure. (Infinitive)

Person of a Verb

Like pronouns, verbs also have first, second, and third person. Person helps determine whether the subject is singular or plural. For example:

	Singular		Plural	
1st person	I	I walk	we	we walk
2nd person	you	you walk	you	you walk
3rd person	he, she, it	he walks	they	they walk

Notice that the third person singular form of the verb *walk* ends in *s*. The verb ends in *s*, but it is not plural. It is singular. The third person verb needs the *s* to make the verb singular. Sometimes the English language does strange things.

Number of a Verb

Verbs, like nouns and pronouns, also have a number. Number indicates whether the verb is singular or plural. The verb must agree in number and person with the subject. If the subject is plural, the verb must be plural; if the subject is singular, the verb must be singular. The relationship between the subject and the verb forms the core of any sentence.

Examples

The *pharmacy* is conveniently located. [*Pharmacy* is singular. The verb *is* is singular.]

A *child dreams* many things when she is young.

Children dream many things when they are young.

Dr. Villmarie and *Dr. Archie operate* together.

Dr. Villmarie also *operates* alone.

Dr. Archie doesn't care to work long hours.

They have too many patients.

Lorry evaluated the problem.

Students work hard on their projects.

Janet works harder on her anatomy than on medical terminology.

Sometimes a group of words separate the subject from the verb, but number agreement between the subject and verb must be maintained.

Examples

The *hygienists* in the office next to the garden *examine* teeth.

Joe, with the extra hours, *accumulated* vacation time.

A compound subject (two or more words joined by *and*) requires a plural verb.

Examples

The *stethoscope and reflex hammer* are tools of the physician.

Jeff and Lorry make good salaries.

When two subjects are combined by *either. . . or, neither. . . nor, not only. . . but also,* the verb agrees with the subject closest to it.

Examples

Neither Janet nor her *sister likes* to give injections.

Neither Janet nor her *sisters like* to give injections.

Not only John but also his *mother lives* near the medical office.

Not only John but also his *parents live* near the medical office.

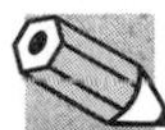

Practice 3-4

Identify the subject in each sentence and select the correct verb from within the parentheses:

1. Shock (is, are) a serious condition. ____________________
2. Sam and Bill (does, do) want to purchase the office space. ____________________
3. The EMTs (resuscitate, resuscitates) patients. ____________________
4. The dental assistant (sterilize, sterilizes) the instruments. ____________________
5. The doctor (palpate, palpates) the internal organs. ____________________
6. The instruments (need, needs) to be calibrated regularly. ____________________
7. The M.A. (need, needs) a new computer. ____________________
8. Employees (work, works) overtime every week. ____________________
9. The patient's tumor (has, have) impaired many systems. ____________________
10. Neither the physician nor the employees (disclose, discloses) patient information. ____________________

Verb Tenses

Verbs in the English language have many tenses (see Figures 3-1 through 3-4). This chapter covers only three: past, present, and future. These are the tenses used most frequently in the allied health setting.

Present Tense

Present tense expresses action that is happening at the *present* time, or action that happens regularly.

Examples

You *work* in a doctor's office.

The doctor *sutures* the laceration in the ER.

The doctor *examines* the patients.

	Meaning	How Formed	Examples: Singular	Examples: Plural	Use in Sentence
Present	Action happens now and regularly	Use main verb	I work You work He, she, it works	We work You work They work	I work 35 hours a week now.
Past	Action begins and ends in the past	Add *d* or *ed* to the main verb	I worked You worked He, she, it worked	We worked You worked They worked	I worked 30 hours a week last year.
Future	Action will occur sometime in the future	Add *will* to the main verb	I will work You will work He, she, it will work	We will work You will work They will work	I will work 40 hours a week next year.

Figure 3-1 Simple Tense

Past Tense

Past tense expresses action that is completed in the past. Notice that *ed* is used to form the past tense of the regular verbs in the examples.

Examples

You *worked* in a doctor's office.

The doctor *sutured* the laceration in the ER.

The doctor *examined* the patients.

	Meaning	How Formed	Examples: Singular	Examples: Plural	Use in Sentence
Present perfect	Started and recently completed	*Have* or *has* + the past participle	I have worked You have worked He, she, it has worked	We have worked You have worked They have worked	I have worked on that project before.
Past perfect	Action finished before another past action	*Had* + the past participle	I had worked You had worked He, she, it had worked	We had worked You had worked They had worked	I had worked on that project when they arrived.
Future perfect	Action finished before another time in the future	*Will have* + the past participle	I will have worked You will have worked He, she, it will have worked	We will have worked You will have worked They will have worked	I will have already worked the new job when the boss arrives.

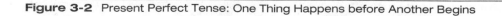

Figure 3-2 Present Perfect Tense: One Thing Happens before Another Begins

	Meaning	How Formed	Examples: Singular	Examples: Plural	Use in Sentence
Present progressive	Action in progress at present and may continue	*Being + ing* to form the present participle	I am working You are working He, she, it is working	We are working You are working They are working	I am working on a book right now.
Past progressive	Action was in progress at a time in the past	*Was + ing*	I was working You were working He, she, it was working	We are working You are working They are working	He was working when I entered the room.
Future progressive	Action will be in progress at a particular time in the future	*Will be + ing*	I will be working You will be working He, she, it will be working	We will be working You will be working They will be working	He will be working when the program begins.

Figure 3-3 Progressive Tense: Action in Progress during a Particular Time

Future Tense

The future tense expresses action that will take place any time after now. To form the future tense, the word *will* is used with the main verb. *Will* is the sign of the future tense.

Examples

You *will work* in a doctor's office

The doctor *will suture* the laceration in the ER.

The doctor *will examine* the patients.

	Meaning	How Formed	Examples: Singular	Examples: Plural	Use in Sentence
Present perfect progressive	Action in progress before now and up to now	*Have, has + been + ing* (present participle)	I have been working You have been working He, she, it has been working	We have been working You have been working They have been working	I have been working for 12 straight hours.
Past perfect progressive	Action in progress before another action in the past	*Had + been + ing*	I had been working You have been working He, she, it will have been working	We had been working You had been working They will have been working	I had been working for 12 hours before I was painting.
Future perfect progressive	Action in progress before an action in the future	*Will have + been + ing*	I will have been working You will have been working He, she, it will have been working	We will have been working You will have been working They will have been working	I will have been working for 12 hours by the time the plant closes.

Figure 3-4 Perfect Progressive Tense: Action in Progress before and up to Another Action

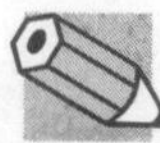

Practice 3-5

Identify the verbs and state whether they are in the past, present, or future tense:

1. The medical assistant wrote "canceled" across the appointment. ________________
2. The physician decides on the most efficient scheduling policy. ________________
3. I will plan on attending the conference. ________________
4. The cancer originated in the lungs. ________________
5. Blood circulates through the body in one minute. ________________
6. The surgeon resected the diseased colon. ________________
7. According to the doctor's testimony, three people witnessed the birth. ________________
8. The patient controls the pain with analgesics. ________________
9. Results of the health survey will be published. ________________
10. Please describe the pain. ________________

Principal Parts of Verbs

As a noun and in connection with grammar, the word *tense* means *time*. Verb tenses tell when an action or state of being occurs. Every verb has four principal parts for denoting tense: the present, past, past participle, and present participle. How verb forms change from one principal part to another categorizes them as regular or irregular verbs.

Regular Verbs

The past tense of regular verbs is formed by adding the letters *d* or *ed* to the present form of the verb. A helping verb is added to the *past* form of the verb to make a *past participle.* Adding *ing* to the present tense forms the present participle.

Examples

Present	*Past*	*Past Participle*	*Present Participle*
introduce	introduced	has, had, have introduced	introducing
look	looked	has, had, have looked	looking
tolerate	tolerated	has, had, have tolerated	tolerating

diagnose	diagnosed	had diagnosed	diagnosing
compare	compared	have compared	comparing
drop	dropped	has dropped	dropping
perform	performed	has performed	performing

Notice that some regular verbs change their spelling to form the past tense or present participle. The rules shown in Figures 3-5 and 3-6 can help make the spelling easier.

1. Verbs ending in *e* drop the *e* and add *ed*: *hope, hoped.*
2. One-syllable verbs ending in a consonant: preceded by one vowel double the final consonant and add *ed*: *stop, stopped*; preceded by two vowels add *ed*: *rain, rained.*
3. Two-syllable verbs ending in a consonant: with the accent on the first syllable add *ed*: *open, opened*; with the accent on the second syllable double the final consonant and add *ed*: *recur, recurred.*
4. Verbs ending in two consonants add *ed*: *start, started.*
5. Verbs ending in *y*: preceded by a vowel keep the *y* and add *ed*: *pray, prayed*; preceded by a consonant change *y* to *i* and add *ed*: *try, tried.*
6. Verbs ending in *ie* add *d*: *lie, lied.*

Figure 3-5 Rules for Forming the Past Tense of Regular Verbs

1. Verbs ending in *e* drop the *e* and add *ing*: *hope, hoping.*
2. One-syllable verbs ending in a consonant: preceded by one vowel double the final consonant and add *ing*: *stop, stopping*; preceded by two vowels add *ing*: *rain, raining.*
3. Two-syllable verbs ending in a consonant with the accent on the first syllable add *ing*: *open, opening*; with the accent on the second syllable double the final consonant and add *ing*: *recur, recurring.*
4. Verbs ending in two consonants add *ing*: *start* to *starting.*
5. Verbs ending in *y*: preceded by a vowel keep the *y* and add *ing*: *pray, praying*; preceded by a consonant keep the *y* and add *ing*: *try, trying.*
6. Verbs ending in *ie* change the *ie* to *y* and add *ing*: *lie, lying.*

Figure 3-6 Rules for Forming the Present Participle of Regular Verbs

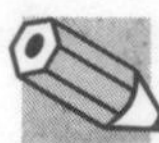

Practice 3-6

Form the present participle, past, and past participle of these regular verbs:

1. accumulate ________ ________ ________
2. elicit ________ ________ ________
3. reveal ________ ________ ________
4. bifurcate ________ ________ ________
5. palpate ________ ________ ________
6. operate ________ ________ ________
7. circulate ________ ________ ________
8. examine ________ ________ ________
9. refer ________ ________ ________
10. suture ________ ________ ________

Irregular Verbs

Only regular verbs follow the rule to add *d* or *ed* to form the past. Many verbs in the English language do not follow this rule. The verbs that do not are called irregular verbs.

Some irregular verbs keep the same form in all four parts:

Present	***Past***	***Past Participle***	***Present Participle***
burst	burst	had burst	bursting
cost	cost	had cost	costing
let	let	had let	letting
set	set	have set	setting
hit	hit	had hit	hitting
read	read	has read	reading
put	put	had put	putting
hurt	hurt	has hurt	hurting

Some irregular verbs change form only once:

Present	***Past***	***Past Participle***	***Present Participle***
cat	eaten	had eaten	eating
sleep	slept	had slept	sleeping
say	said	had said	saying
buy	bought	bought	buying
have	had	had	having
find	found	found	finding

Some irregular verbs change three forms:

Present	***Past***	***Past Participle***	***Present Participle***
tear	tore	had torn	tearing
throw	threw	had thrown	throwing
break	broke	had broken	breaking
drink	drank	drunk	drinking
forgive	forgave	forgiven	forgiving
speak	spoke	spoken	speaking

Many errors are made using irregular verbs. Try to memorize as many principal parts of irregular verbs as possible. See Figure 3-4 for the more commonly encountered irregular verb forms.

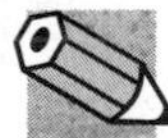

Practice 3-7

Select the correct verb form from within the parentheses:

1. The doctor (dictate, dictated) the operative report.
2. The movement (elicit, elicited) the symptoms.
3. I had (spoke, spoken) to the nurse about the change.
4. The doctor has (flied, flown) to a burn center.
5. The symptoms (occur, occurred) as a result of inadequate circulation.
6. The patient's ankles were (swell, swollen) from edema.

Simple Present	Past	Past Participle	Simple Present	Past	Past Participle
am awake	was awoke	were awoken	know	knew	known
be	was/were	been	leave	left	left
beat	beat	beat	lose	lost	lost
begin	began	begun	make	made	made
bend	bent	bent	prove	proved	proven
bite	bit	bitten	ring	rang	rung
blows	blew	blown	run	ran	run
bring	brought	brought	see	saw	seen
burst	burst	burst	send	sent	sent
catch	caught	caught	sew	sewed	sewn
choose	chose	chosen	shake	shook	shaken
come	came	come	show	showed	shown
cost	cost	cost	shut	shut	shut
cut	cut	cut	sing	sang	sung
do	did	done	sit	sat	sat
draw	drew	drawn	slay	slew	slain
drive	drove	driven	slit	slit	slit
fall	fell	fallen	speak	spoke	spoken
feed	fed	fed	spread	spread	spread
fight	fought	fought	spring	sprang	sprung
flee	fled	fled	steal	stole	stolen
fly	flew	flown	strive	strove	striven
find	found	found	swell	swelled	swollen
forget	forgot	forgotten	swim	swam	swum
freeze	froze	frozen	take	took	taken
get	got	gotten	tear	torn	torn
give	gave	given	throw	threw	thrown
go	went	gone	wake	woke	waken
grew	grown	grown	wear	wore	worn
hang	hang	hung	wring	wrung	wrung
hide	hid	hidden	write	wrote	written
hold	held	held			

Figure 3-7 Past and Past Participle Forms of Common Irregular Verbs

7. Before the shift (begin, began), the nurses (eat, ate, eaten) their lunch.

8. I (came, come) to the ER for help.

9. The driver had (drive, drove, driven) the ambulance right up to the door.

10. The nurse (shook, shake, shaken) the bottle to mix the medication.

Confusing and Troublesome Verbs

Some verbs are frequently confused with verbs that seem to mean the same thing. Even coming up with the correct forms for their principal parts can be troublesome. Errors are made frequently with these verbs, both orally and written. A brief explanation may be helpful.

Lie and Lay

Lie means "recline, rest or stay," as in: "I need to *lie* down for a while." *Lay* means "put or place," as in: "*Lay* your head on the pillow." Here are the principal parts of those two verbs:

Present	*Past*	*Past Participle*	*Present Participle*
lie	lay	lain	lying (reclining)
lay	laid	laid	laying (placing)

Examples

I *lay* the book on the table.

I *lie* down.

I *lay* down yesterday.

I *have lain* down.

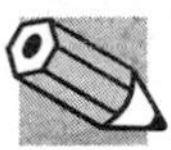

Practice 3-8

Fill in the correct form of the verb lie *or* lay *and state whether the action is to recline or to place:*

1. She has ________________ in bed all day. ________________
2. Joanne ________________ out her clothes before she ________________ down to sleep. ________________
3. The sick patient ________________ ill for days. ________________
4. The M.A. had ________________ the instruments out for the procedure. ________________
5. Where did I ________________ my lab coat? ________________
6. Where have you ________________ it? ________________
7. The letter ________________ on the table all week. ________________
8. I ________________ down when I don't feel well. ________________
9. The medications were ________________ on the table. ________________
10. She was ________________ down when the doctor arrived. ________________

Rise and Raise

Rise means "to move upward by itself or to get up," as in: "Temperatures *rise* in the afternoon." *Raise* means "to lift to a higher position," as in: "*Raise* the cost of medicine by 2 percent." Here are the principal parts of these two verbs:

Present	Past	Past Participle	Present Participle
rise	rose	has risen	rising
raise	raised	had raised	raising

Examples

We *raised* the treatment table an inch higher.

Medical costs *rise.*

Costs *rose* frequently last year.

Costs have *risen.*

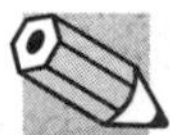

Practice 3-9

Fill in the correct form of the verbs rise or raise: State whether the action is to lift to a higher position, to move upward by itself, or to get up.

1. Hospital costs ___________________ over the previous year.
2. Did the patient's diet ___________________ the blood chemistry levels?
3. The potassium has ___________________ to normal levels.
4. The patient did not ___________________ enough sputum for the test.
5. We had ___________________ early for surgery.
6. Elevated cholesterol in the blood ___________________ the risk of coronary disease.
7. They ___________________ the level of medication needed for the test.
8. Patients ___________________ the issue about high copayments.
9. The committee ___________________ over a million dollars.
10. Patients usually ___________________ about 6:30 a.m.

The key distinction between *lie/lay* and *rise/raise* is that *lay* and *raise* are transitive (the sentence has a direct object) and *lie* and *rise* are intransitive (the sentence has no object).

May and Can

Errors are often made between the words *may* and *can*. *May* means permission or a degree of certainty. To use the word *may* is considered polite.

Examples

You *may* leave at 4:30 p.m. [permission]

May I please borrow your pen? [permission]

The report *may* be true. [degree of certainty]

Can means an ability or a possibility because certain conditions exist.

Examples

You *can* see the wrinkles in the paper. [ability]

A puncture wound *can* cause tetanus. [ability]

I *can* perform the procedure if I get back on time. [possibility]

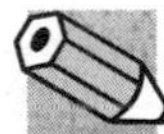

Practice 3-10

Select the correct word from within the parentheses:

1. Call me if you think I (can, may) be of any help.
2. The doctor (can, may) perform that type of operation.
3. Bob and I (may, can) take time off if I (may, can) get someone to take his place.
4. The decision (may, can) affect a lot of staff.
5. You (may, can) do anything you want.
6. The window (can, may) open from the top or the bottom.
7. I (may, can) work on the lab report if you (can, may) find the statistical data.
8. (Can, May) I pick up the Red Cross package now?
9. The phone (may, can) ring off the hook.
10. (Can, May) you complete the article in two weeks?

Use of Verb Tenses in Sentences

Verb tenses express the time of action. Errors arise when the time element in different parts of a sentence does not agree. For example, the use of verb tense in the following sentence is incorrect:

When we *are tired*, we *rested* at the hotel.

The sentence starts in the present tense, *when we are tired*, but according to the rest of the sentence the present action is complete in the past, *we rested at the hotel.* An action begun in the present cannot be completed in the past because it has not occurred yet. The sentence should read:

When we *are tired*, we *rest* at the hotel.

Similarly:

When Valerie *was* young, she likes to *visit* her grandmother. [incorrect]

When Valerie *was* young she *liked* to visit her grandmother. [correct]

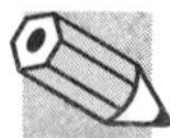

Practice 3-11

Correct the verb tenses in these sentences:

1. The doctor will read the chart before he saw the patient. ____________________
2. If she is smart, she asked for a consultation. ____________________
3. Time flew quickly while we had cleaned the storage closet. ____________________
4. We heard the crash, so we expect an accident. ____________________
5. The family is praying for the patient and will want to show their appreciation. ____________________
6. As the mother was reading, the child is falling asleep. ____________________
7. I would schedule an appointment if I have better insurance. ____________________
8. Aseptic hand washing is crucial if we wanted to prevent transmission of pathogens. ____________________
9. After the rain, the sun come out. ____________________
10. Some people are happy when they felt well. ____________________

Voices of Verbs

Voice shows whether the subject of the verb is doing the action or receiving the action.

Active and Passive Verbs

Verbs have two voices: active and passive. If the subject is doing the action, the verb is in the active voice. If the subject is receiving the action, the verb is passive.

Example	*Voice*	*Explanation*
Bob mailed the letter.	Active	*Bob,* the subject of the sentence, performs the action of the verb *mailed.* The subject, *Bob,* is busy and *actively* in motion.
The letter was mailed by Bob.	Passive	The subject, *letter,* is the receiver of the action of the verb, *mailed.* The subject of the sentence *passively* receives the action.

Examples

John typed three reports a day. [active]

Three reports were typed by John. [passive]

The doctor disclosed the information. [active]

The information was disclosed by the doctor. [passive]

The students transmitted the disease. [active]

The disease was transmitted by the students. [passive]

The surgeon resected the tumor. [active]

The tumor was resected by the surgeon. [passive]

Compare the active and passive voices in the previous sentences. Which voice is heard more often when people speak? Which voice seems easier to speak and understand? Most grammarians agree that the active voice is easier to understand and has more energy. The active voice quickly tells who did what, not what was done by whom. Though grammatically correct, the passive voice lacks strength and clarity. For this reason, writers are encouraged to use the active voice instead of the passive voice. Writers who check their grammar on the computer discover that the computer also frowns on the use of the passive voice.

Identifying the Passive Voice

Since the passive voice should be avoided, how can it be identified? Two elements are clues for detecting the passive voice: (1) a being verb and (2) a past participle. Another signal is the frequent appearance of the word *by* in sentences using the passive voice.

Examples

Three reports a day *were* [being verb] *typed* [past participle] *by* John.

The information *was* [being verb] *disclosed* [past participle] *by* the doctor.

The disease *was* [being verb] *transmitted* [past participle] *by* the students.

Water *was drunk by* the thirsty patients.

Since the use of passive voice is discouraged, it can be changed to the active voice simply by making the direct object the subject. In the passive sentence: "Water was drunk by the *patients*," the direct object is *patients*. Make it the subject of the sentence to achieve active voice: "*Patients* drank the water."

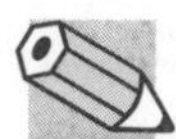

Practice 3-12

Identify the voice as active or passive. If passive, change to active.

1. The conditions are complicated by isolation precautions. ____________________
2. The medication was taken by the patients. ____________________
3. The treatment rooms are cleaned by the people who use them. ____________________
4. The report was read by the surgical team. ____________________
5. Dr. Chris wrote the consult. ____________________
6. The nasogastric tube was used because the patient had esophageal sphincter problems. ____________________
7. The vice president advised cost-cutting procedures. ____________________
8. Dr. Pam biopsied the growth. ____________________
9. The diet was kept by the patient all year. ____________________
10. The surgery began promptly at 7 a.m. ____________________

Moods of Verbs

Mood is the manner in which the action of the sentence is performed. Mood depends on the attitude of the speaker or writer and the purpose of the sentence. Verbs have three moods: indicative, imperative, and subjunctive.

The purpose of the indicative mood is to state a fact or ask a question.

Example

The medical assistant types reports.

The purpose of the imperative mood is to give instruction or commands, or to make requests. The subject of verbs in the imperative mood is always *you*, the person to whom the order is given. The *you* is often omitted from the sentence.

Example

Type this report.

The purpose of the subjunctive mood is to express a command, preference, strong request, or a condition contrary to fact. The subjunctive is formed in two ways: (1) by substituting *be* in place of *am, are,* or *is,* and (2) by dropping the *s* ending from the third person singular, present tense verb.

Example

The doctor requests that her report *be* typed within 24 hours.

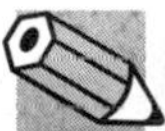

Practice 3-13

Indicate whether the verbs are in the indicative, imperative, or subjunctive mood:

1. We urge that the doctor be given a second chance. ____________________
2. Heart disease is the leading cause of death. ____________________
3. Please remove the soiled linens immediately. ____________________
4. The cardiologist insisted that the EKG be done again. ____________________
5. If I were you, I'd say nothing. ____________________
6. Tell the nurses to be in room five STAT. ____________________
7. Tell the family to be present for the meeting. ____________________
8. Will we be able to cover all patients on the floor? ____________________
9. The hospital has no plans to build a new wing. ____________________
10. Tell the people in the lab that the blood tests must be done today. ____________________

Medical Spelling

Become familiar with the spelling of the following words:

accompany	calibrate
accumulate	circulate
administer	complicate
bifurcate	complains

compose	palpate
diagnose	perform
deteriorate	pulsate
deviate	puncture
disclose	radiate
elicit	recur, recurred, recurrence
evaluate	refer
examine	resect
incubate	resuscitate
introduce	reveals
intubate	stabilize
irrigate	sterilize
ligate	stimulate
occur, occurrence	suture
originate	tolerate
operate	transmit

Verbs Study Summary

Action verb	Expresses both physical and mental activity.	The doctor *operates* on patients. The patient *thought* he was in good health.
Being verb	Any form of the verb to be: *am, is, are, was, were, have, has, had, be, been.*	Erythromycin *is* the cure for bacterial pnuemonia.
Main verb	A single verb in a sentence.	The x-ray *revealed* a fracture in the arm.
Helping verb	A verb that accompanies the main verb: *being verbs, do, shall, will, would, could, can, may, should, must.*	The x-ray *may reveal* a fracture. Many *do believe* that disease is curable.
Linking verb	Connects a compliment: (predicate noun, pronoun, adjective).	The students *felt comfortable* about the changes.
	Common linking verbs: *being verbs, grow, seem, appear, stay, taste.*	The patient *appears* self-motivated. The diet *can include* solids.
Transitive verb	Shows action and needs to complete its meaning.	You must remove the *sutures.*

Intransitive verb	A verb that has no object to receive the action.	The medical report is filed.
Verbals	Verbs that function as nouns, adjectives, adverbs, gerunds (ing + verb), or infinitives (to + verb).	The doctor is *operating*. The doctor wants *to operate*.
Person of a verb	Person speaking (first).	*I* love my medical terminology course. (singular)
	Person spoken to (second).	Do *you* need more medication? (singular or plural)
	Person spoken about (third).	*They* formed an ethics team. (plural)
Number of verb	Indicates singular or plural.	
Verb tenses		
Present	Action happening now.	The nurse works now.
Past	Action completed in the past.	The nurse worked yesterday.
Future	Action will happen later.	The nurse will work tomorrow.

See chapter figures for explanation of additional tenses.

Principle parts of speech.

Regular:		
Past	Forms the past by adding *e* or *ed* to the *present* form of the verb (cure + d = cured).	The doctor *cured* the patient.
Past participle	Add a *helping verb* to form the *past* form (had + cured = had cured).	The doctor *had cured* the patient.
Present participle	Add *ing* to the *present* form of the verb (Cure + ing = curing).	*Curing* patients is the purpose of medicine.
Irregular:		
Past	came	The message *came* by telephone.
Past participle	had come	He *had come* to the end of the paragraph.
Present participle	coming	I'm *coming* to that conclusion.
Voices of verbs:	Shows whether the subject does the action or receives the action.	
Active	The subject does the actions.	The *doctor* made the incision.
Passive	The subject receives the action.	The *incision* was made by the doctor.
Moods of verbs	The manner in which verbs are expressed.	
Indicative	States a fact or asks a question.	Medical examinations are expensive.

Imperative	Makes a request, gives a command or instruction (subject is always the word you).	(you) Take these instruments and sterilize them.
Subjunctive	Expresses a command, preference, strong request, or condition contrary to fact.	The patient must exhaust all other treatments before undergoing chemotherapy.

Skills Review

Following the completed example given as item 1, fill in the missing part of each verb. In the fourth column, state if the verb is regular or irregular.

	Present Tense	Past Tense	Past Participle	Regular/ Irregular
1.	write	wrote	was written	irregular
2.	operate		was operated	
3.		ran	have run	
4.	see	seen		
5.	go		have gone	
6.	fall			
7.		cared		
8.			have diagnosed	
9.	take	took		
10.		dictated		
11.	drive		have driven	
12.	clean		have cleaned	
13.		published		
14.	sterilize		had sterilized	
15.		rained		
16.			had ended	
17.	show			
18.			cost	

19.			has loved
20.	sleep		
21.		sent	
22.			has hurt
23.	say		
24.		read	
25.	finish		was finished

Circle the correct word from within the parenthesis:

First impressions are lasting impressions. Health-care professionals help (project, projects) a positive image to all people (who, whom) they encounter in the medical environment. Medical assistants with a good appearance (has, have) an effect on the patients they (meet, met) daily. The impression that a medical assistant (portrays, portray) to the patients (color, colors) the image of the physician and the care the patients expect.

Good grooming is essential in fostering good impressions. Good grooming (include, includes) a bath or shower daily, use of deodorant, and good oral hygiene. Hair should be (clean, cleaned), neatly styled, and above the collar. Shoes should be comfortable. Laces in shoes (need, needs) to be washed often.

The usual attire in the medical setting (is, are) uniforms, depending on the dress code of the medical facility. A uniform (give, gives) the impression of professionalism and (identify, identifies) the person as a member of the health-care team. Wear a clean uniform to work daily. In offices where a uniform is not (required, requires), the medical assistant is expected to show good taste in selecting and wearing a professional wardrobe.

The amount of jewelry (is, are) limited to an engagement ring, wedding band, or professional pin. Sometimes staff members (wear, wears) name tags to help patients (identify, identifies) the health-care provider by name.

A frequent problem that (surface, surfaces) with health-care workers (is, are) burnout. Medical assistants need to take care of (himself, herself, themselves). Good health habits (include, includes) frequent exercise, eight hours of sleep each night, and eating the right kinds of food.

Good appearance and good health habits (is, are) important habits to foster in health-care professionals.

Correctly rewrite the italicized word above the error:

The law maintains that each physician is responsible for *their* own negligence when someone is injured. A physician is also responsible for the negligent act *performs* by medical assistants employed in *their* office. An injured party generally *sue* the doctor because there is a better chance of collecting more money. A medical assistant is not licensed to practice medicine. One must be careful what he or she *discuss* with the patient. Patients may think the medical *assistants* remarks as those of the physician. These facts *illustrates* the importance of performing all actions with extreme care.

Identify the verbs in the following sentences as transitive or intransitive:

1. The doctor hired an attorney to settle the claim. ____________________
2. The lawyer arrived late for the meeting. ____________________
3. The judge appeared impatient. ____________________
4. The lawyer presented his case to the judge. ____________________
5. The judge ruled in favor of the patient. ____________________

Circle the verb phrase in each sentence:

1. The decision was made.
2. By the end of this year, the book will have been printed.
3. Each new employee is required to have a physical.
4. Many patients are fearful and tense.
5. Hypertension has been called the silent disease.

Circle the correct verb from within the parentheses:

1. Everyone in the hospital (know, knows) Doreen is the best nurse.
2. Patients (appreciate, appreciates) good health care.
3. When I went to the hospital, I was (took, take, taken) to the emergency room.

4. The problem (is, are) we have no empty beds.

5. A young or older person (make, makes) choices in life.

6. Two weeks after the operation, the patient (file, files, filed) a complaint.

7. After the lecture, the nurse (ran, run) to her appointment.

8. By June, they will have (pay, paid, payed) the balance of the cost.

9. The food (lie, lay) on the tray, untouched.

10. I (caught, catched) the flu while visiting relatives in New England.

11. The patient (sat, sit, set) in the chair.

12. Yesterday the patient (drink, drank, drunk) eight glasses of water.

13. Six people (were hurt, has hurt, was hurting) in the accident.

14. A vial of blood was (draw, drew, drawn) from the patient.

15. The man was (give, gave, given) assistance to get into the wheelchair.

16. The doctor's practice (grew, grow, grown) quickly.

17. Most people with cancer (fight, fought) for life.

18. The next patient to be (see, saw, seen) is a young child.

19. Did you (do, did, done) a thorough physical on this man?

20. The man had (lie, lay, lain) in bed for three days before calling a doctor.

Simplify these sentences correctly:

1. Sutures came in a variety of materials such as silk and catgut which is from sheep's intestines.

   ____

2. The type of sutures which the surgeon ties each stitch separately is called interrupted.

   ____

3. The diameter (gauge) of the suture material vary from fine (11-0) to very coarse (3).

___

4. The 6-0 suture is also called six aught and might be wrote 000000. It is very fine.

___

5. Whole numbers such as 1, 2, 3, and 4 imply that the suture is very large diameter thread. This is very coarse suture material.

___

Circle the correct spelling in each line:

1. punchered	resucitate	sterilised	radiate
2. biforcate	pulsat	stabilised	irrigate
3. reconect	irigate	examine	operatted
4. transmitted	transmited	transmmitted	trannsmitted
5. incubatte	circulate	refferred	imapairr
6. diviate	deveate	deviate	deviatte
7. acompanied	accompannied	acomppanied	accompanied
8. vomet	originate	irigate	reconect
9. diteriorate	detteriorate	deteriorate	detereorat
10. examine	acumulate	administir	desclose

Translate medical abbreviations using a medical dictionary or appendix.

1. DPT ___
2. Dx ___
3. EEG ___
4. DRGs ___

5. DO ___________________

6. EOM ___________________

7. FBS ___________________

8. F.U.O ___________________

9. F/U ___________________

10. Fx ___________________

Chapter 4

Adjectives

Objectives

Upon completion of this chapter, the student should be able to:

- recognize and understand various types of adjectives
- be aware of adjective placement to ensure clearer sentences
- recognize suffixes that form descriptive adjectives
- use adjectives to make comparisons
- spell various medical terms
- translate various medical abbreviations
- recognize sentences that contain misplaced modifiers
- understand the use of eponyms in medical documentation

Types of Adjectives

In the first three chapters, three important parts of speech were explained: nouns, pronouns, and verbs. These words are important because the noun (or pronoun, which takes the place of a noun) and verb constitute the main part of a sentence. A sentence must have a noun or implied pronoun (*you*) as the subject and a verb in order to express a complete thought, otherwise there is no sentence. However, additional words or parts of speech are used to make sentences clearer and more enjoyable to read and write. These additional words—adjectives and adverbs—complement, describe, add meaning to, or explain the noun and verb (Figure 4-1).

Noun	Verb	Additional Clarifying Words
Nurses	observe	Nurses observe *reactions to treatments.*
Doctors	operate	Doctors operate in *emergency situations.*
He	speaks	He speaks *with authority about accreditation.*
M.A.s	transcribe	M.A.s transcribe *medical reports*

Figure 4-1 Adding Meaning to Sentences

This chapter explains the part of speech called an adjective. (Adverbs are covered in Chapter 5.) An adjective is a word that describes a noun or pronoun. It changes the meaning of the noun by giving more information about it. In the sentences that follow, notice how the adjectives further clarify the nouns they modify:

The *new* members of the team will arrive next week.

The doctor gives a *thorough* examination.

Hospital policies often require *legal* consultation.

These grades show knowledge of *body* systems.

Your *license* renewal is due *this* month.

Limiting Adjectives

Adjectives describe four important facts about nouns and pronouns by answering the questions *which one? how many? how much?* and *what kind?* Adjectives that answer the first three questions are called limiting adjectives because they limit the nouns to a definite or indefinite amount. Common limiting adjectives are *a, an, all, any, both, each, every, few, many, more, most, much, no, some, such, this, that, these, those, the, one* (or any other number), and *possessive nouns* and *pronouns* used as adjectives.

Examples

some diseases	*two* patients	*this* streptococcal
many meetings	*each* day	*the* myocardial infarction
a necrotic tumor	*an* exam	*my* medication
our office	*your* license	*their* medical records

All pathological findings should be recorded.

These charts are going to the Medical Records Department.

Their system works best for that individual practice.

Adjectives that tell *what kind* are called descriptive adjectives and are covered in the next section.

A and AN

A and *an* are limiting adjectives called indefinite articles. (The word *the* is also an article, a "definite" article.) When deciding between the use of *a* or *an*, consider the sound of the word that follows the article rather than its spelling. The *a* is used before words that begin with a consonant sound, including the sounds *h*, long *u*, and an *o* with the sound of *w* (as in "one"). The word *an* is used before words that begin with a vowel sound.

Examples

a uric acid test [long *u* sound]

a one-day seminar [*w* sound]

an unsuccessful medication [vowel sound]

an honor [because the letter *h* is silent, the word begins with a vowel sound]

an abdominal incision [vowel sound]

a cross-section	*a* uniform	*an* asset
an antidiuretic pill	*an* inguinal hernia	*an* eight-hour day
an outcome	*an* x-ray reading	

Singular and Plural

A limiting adjective must agree with the noun or pronoun it limits. Limiting adjectives used with singular nouns are *a, an, each, every, either, this, that, neither,* and *one.*

Examples

an order	*either* instrument	*neither* doctor	*one* calculus
every patient	*this* bed	*every* report	*each* stitch

Limiting adjectives used with plural nouns are *few, several, many, these, those,* and *two* (or any number other than one).

Examples

These reports need to be filed tomorrow.

Several reports must be transcribed by tomorrow morning.

The limiting adjectives *all, any,* and *some* can be either singular or plural.

all data   *some* information   *any* problems

Some limiting adjectives may change into other parts of speech, depending on how they are used in a sentence. One example is the adjective *many.* It can be used as an adjective or a pronoun. If the word modifies a noun or pronoun, it is an adjective. If the word functions alone as a subject, direct object, indirect object, or object of a preposition, it is a pronoun.

Examples

Limiting Adjective	*Many* medical assistants are taking the certification exam. [*Many* describes the noun *assistants* and is used as an adjective.]
Pronoun	*Many* of the medical assistants are taking the certification exam. [*Many* is used alone as a subject pronoun.]

Interrogative and Proper Adjectives

Two limiting adjectives, *which* and *what,* are called interrogative adjectives because they ask *direct* or *indirect* questions. In the first case, a question is asked directly by the person wanting the answer. An additional step is added with the *indirect* question. The question is asked for someone else. *Which* is used when the speaker wants someone to make a choice among alternatives.

Examples

Direct Questions	*What* time is it, Bill?
	Which room is available for the patient?
Indirect Questions	The nurse wants to know *which* hours she will be working.
	The nurse wants to know *what* time the doctor is expected.

A proper adjective has its source within a proper noun, such as the word *Italian*, which comes from the proper noun *Italy*. Like the proper noun, the proper adjective begins with a capital letter.

Italian spaghetti   *Spanish* influence   *American* citizen

Eponyms are also proper adjectives. An eponym comes from the surname of a person after which something is named, as in *Foley* catheter or *Mayo* scissors. Because eponyms are so important in medical documentation, more information is provided in a separate section later in this chapter.

Predicate and Compound Adjectives

Adjectives may also be used as predicate adjectives. Like their noun counterparts, predicate adjectives come after *being* verbs.

Examples

Smoking is *dangerous* to your health. [*Dangerous* is in the predicate, follows the being verb *is*, and describes the noun *smoking*.]

Health fairs are *educational.*

The word "compound" means to combine two or more elements. Compound adjectives combine two or more describing words that act as a single describer. When the compound adjective comes before the noun it describes, it is usually hyphenated for clarity. When the compound adjective comes after the noun it describes, a hyphen is not usually used.

Examples

The hospital has *state-of-the-art* technology. [before the noun]

The technology at the hospital is *state of the art.* [after the noun]

She had *second-degree* burns on her upper extremities. [before]

The burns on her upper extremities were *second degree.* [after]

A number plus a noun of single measurement (*16-unit*) is hyphenated when it comes before the noun. The number and noun is not hyphenated when it follows a noun.

Examples

The hospital is a *six-story* building.	The hospital has *six stories.*
The *one-inch* wound needed sutures.	The wound with sutures was *one inch.*

Fractions are hyphenated when they are spelled out:

Two-thirds, one-half *Two-thirds* of the faculty were women.

Some frequently used adjectives are not hyphenated because they are considered one word.

childbirth earache nosebleed painless

In a series of adjectives with the same root word, omit all but the last root word.

Examples

Incorrect The medicine will take 5-*bottle*, 10-*bottle*, and 12-*bottle* sizes.

Correct The medicine will take 5-, 10-, and 12-*bottle* sizes.

Correct The report will have a four-to-six-*week* delay.

A comma is placed between two or more adjectives that express different concepts about the noun they describe.

Examples

The *young, polite* intern expressed good bedside manners.

The ambulance was a *large, colorful* vehicle.

The ambulance was a *large, well-equipped* vehicle.

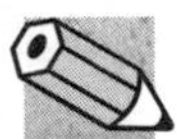

Practice 4-1

Choose the correct limiting adjective from within the parentheses:

1. (Many, a) nurse works on the third floor.
2. (A, An) nurse likes to work on the first shift.
3. (One, Two) elevators are available for ambulatory patients.
4. The doctor ordered (these, this) medications a week ago.
5. (Several, each) alarm goes off when the door is opened.
6. Employees were asked to select (a, an) dental plan.
7. (Several, One) persons applied for that job.
8. (Most, An) medications are found in the pharmacy.
9. Dr. Williams wants to know the answer to (that, those) problem.
10. The medical assistant completed (each, both) tasks before leaving the office.

Hyphenate the adjectives where necessary.

1. The laboratory uses state of the art technology.
2. The doctor made many off the record comments.
3. Mrs. Archie's medical record is up to date.
4. Ready to wear uniforms are popular with nurses.
5. A well known physician will do the operation.
6. The patient is receiving an in depth series of tests.
7. Well meaning people give the wrong information under pressure.
8. The patient is a well developed, well nourished young man.
9. The ambulance driver was a well trained emergency technician.
10. The medication is to be administered at 3, 6, and 9 hour intervals.

Descriptive Adjectives

Descriptive adjectives modify nouns or pronouns by describing their characteristics or qualities. Descriptive adjectives are perhaps the easiest type of adjective to understand. They provide clarity by adding specifics about the nouns they describe.

Examples

The *tall* nurse wore a *white* uniform.

The *streptococcal* infection spread through the *respiratory* system.

The *medical* assistant took the patient's *medical* history.

Physical assessment is an *essential* aspect of *medical* care.

The *Trendelenburg* position is used in cases of shock, in some *abdominal* surgery, and for patient's with *low blood* pressure.

Many descriptive adjectives have common endings or suffixes:

Ending	***Examples***
able, an, ian	cap*able*, Americ*an*, Canad*ian*, reli*able*
iac	card*iac*, cel*iac*, man*iac*
al, ant, eal, ical	cervic*al*, occipit*al*, or*al*, periton*eal*, patholog*ical*, const*ant*
ar, ary, ent	muscul*ar*, preval*ent*, pulmon*ary*, transi*ent*, independ*ent*

ese, ful	Chin*ese*, wonder*ful*, care*ful*, cheer*ful*
ial	influent*ial*, part*ial*
ible, ic, tic	leg*ible*, chron*ic*, epigastr*ic*, thorac*ic*, necro*tic*, hydrochlor*ic*
ior	infer*ior*, anter*ior*, super*ior*
ive, ly	posit*ive*, friend*ly*, comprehens*ive*, manipulat*ive*
ous	delici*ous*, muc*ous*, anxi*ous*
oid, ose	muc*oid*, epiderm*oid*, adip*ose*
ual, y	punct*ual*, tid*y*, chill*y*

A noun may also be used as an adjective. Nouns become adjectives when they are used to describe other nouns.

Examples

The *uniform* store went out of business. [The noun *uniform* becomes an adjective because it describes the noun *store.*]

The patient's *blood* pressure is rising slowly.

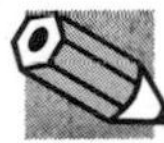

Practice 4-2

Identify the descriptive adjectives in each sentence:

1. The nurse is a likeable and friendly person. ____________________
2. Clinical examination showed external bleeding. ____________________
3. Allied health professionals must be responsible employees. ____________________
4. General procedures should be followed for hospital admission. ____________________
5. Triangular bandages are used in first aid. ____________________
6. Shock is a serious condition. ____________________
7. A comprehensive examination is given to new employees. ____________________
8. Severe coughing can produce asphyxia. ____________________
9. A detailed, clinical evaluation was part of the report. ____________________
10. The ethics board discussed questionable actions by one staff member. ____________________

Placement of Adjectives

The placement of adjectives in a sentence is important to its meaning. To write clearer sentences, place adjectives near the nouns they describe.

- Before the noun: The *doctor's* report was filed correctly. The patient had a *radical* mastectomy.
- After the noun: The report, *exceptional* in detail, provided the necessary information. The doctor, *alert* to physical signs, diagnosed the problem.
- After a linking verb: Just as there is a predicate noun, so, too, there is a predicate adjective. The predicate adjective is found after a being verb and describes a subject noun or pronoun.

  He is apprehensive. [*Apprehensive* describes the subject pronoun *he* and follows the being verb *is*.]

  Shock is *serious*. [*Serious* follows the word *is* and modifies the noun *shock*.]

- At the beginning of a sentence: Alert to *physical* signs, the doctor diagnosed the problem. *Paleness, perspiration,* and *dizziness* are some of the symptoms of this disease.

In a group of adjectives that contains a limiting adjective and one or more descriptive adjectives *that all modify the same noun,* place the limiting adjective first. If there is a noun adjective, it is placed immediately before the noun it modifies; for example:

Limiting Adjective	**Descriptive Adjective**	**Noun Modified**	
The	first aid	classes	begin tomorrow.
That	bleeding gunshot	wound	was an accident.

Misplaced Modifiers

Misplaced modifiers, either words or phrases, can easily result in unintended and sometimes humorous interpretations:

Once a village blacksmith found an apprentice willing to work hard at low pay. The smith immediately began his instructions to the young fellow. "When I take the material out of the fire, I'll lay it on the anvil and when I nod my head, you hit it with the hammer." The apprentice did precisely what he thought he was told. Next day, he was the village blacksmith. (Source Unknown.)

What happens to a sentence when the modifier is misplaced? A different placement of a modifier can completely change the meaning of a sentence.

Examples

The doctor had six patients *only* yesterday.

The doctor *only* had six patients yesterday.

The doctor had six patients yesterday *only*.

Consider these sentences with misplaced modifiers:

Misplaced	A medical assistant almost completed all of her procedures.
Revised	A medical assistant completed almost all of her procedures.
Misplaced	The patient in her peritoneal cavity had fluid accumulations.
Revised	The patient had fluid accumulation in her peritoneal cavity.
Misplaced	An ambulance is parked behind the hospital which is out of emergency I.V. fluid.
Revised	An ambulance, which is out of emergency I.V. fluid, is parked behind the hospital.
Misplaced	Give the head injury the anesthetic.
Revised	Give the anesthetic to the patient with the head injury.
Misplaced	Here are some suggestions to improve your illness from the cardiologist.
Revised	Here are some suggestions from the cardiologist to improve your illness.
Misplaced	Demerol was received by the patient of 100 milligrams intramuscularly for the pain.
Revised	The patient received Demerol, 100 milligrams, intramuscularly for the pain.

Although many misplaced modifiers result in humor, some could have serious consequences, particularly in legal situations. The court often requests medical records in malpractice cases. Sentences open to various interpretations provide a field day in court that could result in high financial loses.

The way to detect misplaced modifiers is to identify them and rearrange them near the word or words they modify. Read the following paragraph and note the possibilities for misinterpretation:

Patient is a 40-year-old, white female who came to the ER with chest pain at 3:30 a.m. (Who came to the ER, the patient or the pain?) *The patient called me stating the chest pain was acute prior to the ER visit.* (Did the patient call the doctor before the visit, or was the pain acute before the visit?) *The pain moving toward the neck was located in the right substernal area.* (Was the pain located in the neck or the right substernal area?) *Now under control with insulin, she has a history of diabetes.* (Is the chest pain or diabetes under control with insulin?) *Her mother died of myocardial infarction at 45.* (Did the infarction die at 45 or the mother?)

Here is the paragraph rewritten for clarity:

The patient is a 40-year-old, white female with chest pain who came to the ER at 3:30 a.m. Prior to the ER visit, the patient called me stating the chest pain was acute. The pain was located in the right substernal area moving toward the neck. She has a history of diabetes now under control with insulin. The patient's mother died at 45 from myocardial infarction.

Practice 4-3

Revise and simplify these sentences:

1. The computer is in Dr. Villa's office that doesn't work. ________________
2. Buy medicine from the pharmacy with a generic brand. ________________
3. The hospital provides comfort for people with central air conditioning. ________________
4. The high doctor was displeased with the temperature reading. ________________
5. The nurse dropped the report I wrote in the wastebasket. ________________
6. He was described as a psychotherapist with multiple problems. ________________
7. Motor vehicle accidents are the leading cause in the United States of death. ________________
8. The appearance in urine is normal of a few epithelial cells. ________________
9. The gift shop sells combs for people with unbreakable teeth. ________________
10. She bought a stethoscope from the medical supply store that was expensive. ________________
11. A well-balanced diet is difficult but rewarding to control weight. ________________
12. Balanced foods to maintain weight are necessary. ________________
13. Medical assistants with rapid changes must keep current. ________________
14. Supervise the patient's registration form completion. ________________
15. One of the doctors for emergencies is available in the group. ________________

Degrees of Adjectives to Express Comparison

Degrees of adjectives help describe the quality of a person, place, thing, or idea in comparison to another person, place, thing, or idea. Because qualities vary, adjectives have three different degrees of comparison: the positive, comparative, and superlative.

Positive

The positive degree describes nouns *without* making a comparison. The adjective is in its *base* form.

Examples

The hospital has *capable* doctors. This report is *good*.

Ms. Archer is a *fast* transcriber. Mr. Oberg is *reliable*.

Comparative

Comparative adjectives compare two persons, places, things, or ideas. They are formed in two ways:

1. Add *r* or *er* to the positive or base form of the word. If the word ends in *y*, change the *y* to *i* and add *er*.

   ### Examples

   young to young*er* fat to fatt*er* tall to tall*er*

   happy to happ*ier* healthy to health*ier* smart to smart*er*

   The operation was *tougher* than the last one.

   This report is *longer* than the pathology report.

   Ms. O'Conner is a *faster* transcriber than the secretary.

2. Add the word *more* or *less* to adjectives of two or more syllables.

   ### Examples

   difficult to *more difficult* successful to *more successful*

   The left ventricle is *more muscular* than the right ventricle.

   The patient's medical record is *more reliable* than this letter.

Some adjectives are irregular. See under "Other Comparisons."

Superlative

Superlative adjectives are used to compare three or more persons, places, things, or ideas. They usually end in *st* or *est* and are formed in two ways:

1. Add *st* or *est* to the base form of a one-syllable adjective and some two-syllable adjectives. If the word ends in *y*, change the *y* to *i* before adding est.

   ### Examples

   This lab report is the *longest* one of all the reports.

   Your appointment is the *earliest* in the day.

2. Insert the word *most* or *least* before the base form of an adjective of two or more syllables.

Examples

Mr. Jones is the *most reliable* medical assistant in the hospital.

The *least important* appointment on the schedule needs to be cancelled.

Dr. Villes is the *most competent* physician in his field.

Some adjectives are irregular. See under "Other Comparisons."
The superlative degree may be used for emphasis when there is no obvious comparison.

As a nurse, you are the *greatest.*

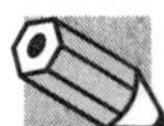

Practice 4-4

Indicate the comparative and superlative degrees of these adjectives:

1. weak ________________ ________________
2. difficult ________________ ________________
3. painful ________________ ________________
4. dry ________________ ________________
5. much ________________ ________________
6. late ________________ ________________
7. hard ________________ ________________
8. far ________________ ________________
9. heavy ________________ ________________
10. thick ________________ ________________
11. irritable ________________ ________________
12. consistent ________________ ________________
13. healthy ________________ ________________
14. visible ________________ ________________
15. comfortable ________________ ________________

16. sick ________________ ________________

17. bad ________________ ________________

18. extensive ________________ ________________

19. early ________________ ________________

20. clean ________________ ________________

Other Comparisons

Some commonly used adjectives are irregular when they form the comparative and superlative degrees:

Positive	***Comparative***	***Superlative***
bad	worse	worst
good	better	best
little	less	least
many/much	more	most

Consult a dictionary if you are unsure about the correct word to use.

One of the most common mistakes made in comparisons is using the *double comparison*, or combining *er* with the base word and using *more,* or combining *est* and using *most.*

Examples

Incorrect	more poorer	most poorest
Correct	poorer or more poor	poorest or most poor

Other common mistakes involve the misuse of the words *than* and *as* when making a comparison. *Than* introduces a second person, place, thing, or idea into the comparison.

Examples

The right arm is less cyanotic *than* the left arm.

Telecommunications is faster *than* sending mail.

In expressing both positive and comparative degrees in one sentence, use the word *as* after the positive adjective and the word *than* after the comparative adjective.

Examples

Your method of filing is *as* well organized, but more complex *than* our method.

The medicine is affordable *as* always, but less expensive *than* the brand name.

Additionally, do not confuse the word *than* with the word *then*. *Than* is used when comparing modifiers. *Then* means *at that time.*

Examples

Your epigastric pain isn't better *than* yesterday's pain?

The incision was made and *then* the retractors were used.

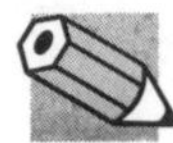

Practice 4-5

Identify the correct comparative degree needed for each sentence:

1. confident — Physicians are __________________ than they were ten years ago.
2. colorful — This hematoma is the __________________ of all your bruises.
3. bad — The peptic ulcer is __________________ than ever.
4. new — This x-ray machine is a __________________ model than the last one.
5. difficult — The comprehensive exam was __________________.
6. low — The height of this file cabinet is __________________ than the one in your office.
7. fast — The __________________ way to the emergency room is up Main Street.
8. great — John is __________________ but Bill is __________________.
9. cheap — The uniform is made of the __________________ material we can find.
10. competent — The intern is __________________, but the specialist is __________________.

Troublesome Adjectives

Some adjectives need special attention in their use.

Farther	Refers to distance or a remote point: "Worcester is *farther* east than Springfield."
Further	Means additional or to a greater extent: "*Further* information is needed before the operation is scheduled."
Later	Refers to the second of two events that occur in chronological order: "The medical assistant reserved a flight *later* in the day."

Latter	Refers to the second of two things presented together: "The doctor could use OR 1 or OR 2, but decided on the latter."
Last	Refers to the final item in a list or series: "The *last* payment is due in January."
Latest	Refers to the most recent of something in chronological order: "The answering machine is the *latest* model produced."
Loose	Means free, not tied to something: "Wear *loose* clothing in a wheelchair."
Lose	Means to part with something unintentionally: "The physician did not want to *lose* his stethoscope."

Eponyms

Eponyms are used frequently in medical documentation. An eponym is the name of something derived from and identified with a real or mythical person. A medical eponym is the real surname of an individual who is connected with a particular treatment, operation, or instrument. It is very important to spell these eponym adjectives correctly. When in doubt about correct spelling, consult a medical dictionary.

Eponyms are capitalized but not the nouns associated with them: Parkinsonism fibers, Bartholin's glands, tetralogy of Fallot, Cheyne-Stokes respirations, Bell's palsy, Babinski's sign, APGAR score, Trendelenburg's position, Epstein-Barr virus, Buck's extension, bundle of His, Fowler's position, DeBakey prosthesis.

Words derived from eponyms need not be capitalized: parkinsonism, fallopian tube, eustachian tubes.

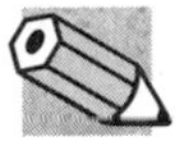

Practice 4-6

Identify the eponyms in each sentence:

1. Adam Smith in the pediatric ward has a tetralogy of Fallot. ____________________
2. What is the newborn's APGAR score at one minute? ____________________
3. Teenagers are sometimes prone to the Epstein-Barr virus. ____________________
4. Place the patient in a semi-Fowler's position. ____________________
5. Bell's palsy may sometimes go away within six months. ____________________
6. Alzheimer's disease is the presence of plaques in the brain. ____________________
7. The Swan-Ganz catheter measures the pressure in the heart. ____________________
8. The Babinski's sign is present in infancy. ____________________
9. Buck's extension is skin traction used to immobilize a limb. ____________________
10. The overhead frame is part of Russell traction. ____________________

Degrees of Comparison

	Degree			
Number of Syllables	**Positive (base, describes without making a comparison)**	**Comparative (compares two or more)**	**Superlative (compares three or more)**	**Rule**
One syllable	young, new, light, healthy	younger , newer, lighter, healthier	youngest, newest, lightest, healthiest	Add *er* or *est* to base. For words ending in *y*, change *y* to *i* and *er* or *est*.
Two of more syllables	gentle, expensive, fascinating	more gentle, more expensive, more fascinating	most gentle, most expensive, most fascinating	Use *more* and *most*.
Irregular adjectives	good	better	best	
	bad	worse	worst	
	little	less	least	
	many	much	most	

Medical Spelling

Become familiar with the spelling of the following words:

abdominal
anterior
antidiuretic
apprehensive
bronchial
calculus, calculi
cyanotic
clinical
comprehensive
dorsal
epithelial
excessive
fetal
frontal
gastrointestinal
hepatic
infection
inguinal
intravenous
lateral
muscular
mucous
myocardial infarction
nasogastric
necrotic
pathological

pelvic	skeletal
peptic ulcer	streptococcal
peritoneal	superficial
pleural	thoracic
proximal	tonsillar
respiratory	uric acid
retractor	urinary

Adjectives Study Summary

Adjective	**Describes a noun or pronoun.**	
Limiting	Limits the noun or pronoun to a definite or indefinite amount. Answers how many, how much, which one.	a, an, all, any, both, each, every, few, many, more, most, much, no, some, such, that, those, this, these, numbers, possessive nouns, and pronouns.
Interrogative	Asks a question	which, what.
Proper	Finds its source in a proper noun.	American citizen. Russian immigrant.
Compound	Combines two or more describing words as a single modifier.	state-of-the-art computer (before noun). The computer is state of the art (after noun). over-crowded bus. 5-,10-, 15- cent stamps.
Predicate	Describes a subject and comes after a being verb.	The needle is *sharp*. The x-rays are *clear*.
Descriptive	Describes the quality of the person, place, thing, or idea of the noun.	red, large, generous, energetic, partial, beautiful, organized, hungry, poetic, powerful.

Skills Review

Identify the adjectives in each sentence:

1. A streptococcal infection is serious. ___________________
2. Protein repairs tissues damaged by disease. ___________________
3. A good trait for a nurse is compassion. ___________________

4. A pathologist studies diseased tissues. ____________________

5. Gangrene is obstruction of blood flow resulting in necrotic tissue. ____________________

6. The patient was taking an antidiuretic medication. ____________________

7. Myocardial infarction is the medical term for heart attack. ____________________

8. The auto accident occurred at midnight. ____________________

9. Gastrointestinal upset is a side effect of many medications. ____________________

10. His headaches originated in the dorsal part of the head. ____________________

Fill in the specific kind of adjective requested on the left.

1. Limiting ____________________ staff members work on weekends.
2. Descriptive Insurance covers only ____________________ benefits.
3. Interrogative ____________________ report do you want faxed?
4. Predicate The hospital logo was ____________________.
5. Proper All ____________________ citizens must have a social security number.
6. Compound The ____________________ letter explained the problem.
7. Interrogative ____________________ day of the week can you work overtime?
8. Descriptive The ____________________ test came back normal.
9. Limiting The nurse scheduled ____________________ appointment for 4:30 p.m.
10. Proper Physicians take the ____________________ oath.

Write medical adjectives having these suffixes:

1. al ____________________
2. ian ____________________
3. ior ____________________
6. ic ____________________
7. ous ____________________
8. ual ____________________

4. able ____________________ 9. iac ____________________

5. cal ____________________ 10. ary ____________________

Circle the correct word within the parentheses in each sentence:

1. Medicine is (most, more) competitive (then, than) it was ten years ago.
2. The hospital is one of the (busy, busier, busiest) facilities in the country.
3. Dr. Ray is (good, better, best) but Dr. Taft is (good, better, best).
4. The medical terminology book (further, farther) explains the meaning of words.
5. Over a period of time, (fewer, less) numbers of people applied for the job.
6. I prefer the (latter, later) document to the first one.
7. The (all-encompassing, all encompassing) remarks were transcribed.
8. The (poor, poorer, poorest) mark in the class was 70%.
9. And (farther, further) more, give up smoking right now.
10. This shipment is the (heavy, heavier, heaviest) one all year.

Write true or false next to the following statements:

1. Adjectives answer what kind and how many. ____________________
2. A noun can be used as an adjective. ____________________
3. The letters *est* are a sign of the comparative degree. ____________________
4. The letters *er* are used to describe three or more persons, places, things, or ideas. ____________________
5. The base word and the positive word mean the same thing. ____________________
6. A hyphen is used in a compound adjective positioned before the noun it modifies. ____________________
7. *This, that, these,* and *those* are examples of descriptive adjectives. ____________________

8. Limiting adjectives can be placed anywhere in a sentence. ____________________

9. To show comparison, the word *most* or *least* is placed before the base form of an adjective of two or more syllables. ____________________

10. When a proper adjective is not associated with a proper noun as its base, no capital letter is needed. ____________________

Grammar Exercise: Underline each error in the paragraph and write its correction above the word.

Based on the evaluation, the patient will be addmitted to the hospital. The patient was placed on a high dose of NSAID. The report concerning the patients abdominal xray were obtained. The patient requiered an intervanous before reaching the hospital. The patients' condition will probably give some pain. This pain can be relieved by over the counter medication. Please call the ofice if there are any questions.

Rewrite these sentences to make them logical:

1. On the second day the knee was better and on the third day it completely disappeared.

   ____

2. The patient left the hospital feeling much better except for her original complaints.

   ____

3. The patient has chest pain if she lies on her left side for over a year.

   ____

4. The patient has been depressed ever since she began seeing me ten years ago.

   ____

5. By the time he was admitted, his rapid heart had stopped and he was feeling better.

   ____

6. She is numb from her toes down.

   ____

7. The patient is tearful and crying constantly. She also appears to be depressed.

   ____

8. When she fainted, her eyes rolled around the room.

___

9. The patient's past medical history has been insignificant with only a 40lb.weight gain in the last three days.

___

10. Mrs. Mongeon had an x-ray that showed pleurisy.

___

Circle the correctly spelled word in each line:

1. bronchal	bronchial	bronkial	branchiol
2. cephelic	cefalic	cephalich	cephalic
3. epithelel	epithelial	epathelial	epathelil
4. gastrointestianl	gastrointistinal	gastrointestinal	gastraintistinal
5. mocous	mucos	mucous	nocous
6. pleural	plueral	pleurel	pluerel
7. streptococcal	streptocaccal	stretococcal	streptocacal
8. comprihensive	conprehensive	comprehensive	comprehinsive
9. urinery	uranary	urenery	urinary
10. pathlogical	pathilogical	pathological	patholgical

Translate medical abbreviations using a medical dictionary or appendix.

1. gtt ___
2. Hct ___
3. hgb ___
4. HPI ___
5. gm ___

6. Hx ____________________

7. I&D ____________________

8. IM ____________________

9. I&O ____________________

10. IVP ____________________

Chapter 5

Adverbs

Objectives *Upon completion of this chapter, the student should be able to:*

- recognize and use adverbs effectively
- distinguish between the use of adjectives and adverbs
- change adjectives into adverbs
- use adverbs to make accurate degrees of comparisons
- avoid the use of double negatives
- place adverbs appropriately
- spell various medical terms
- translate various medical abbreviations

Recognizing Adverbs

Learning about parts of speech may be confusing at times because there are so many exceptions to the rules of grammar. However, some parts of speech have similar characteristics that help simplify understanding of their usage. As mentioned in Chapter 2, pronouns take the place of nouns and are used in many similar ways: as subjects, direct objects, and indirect objects. The same kind of relationship exists between adjectives and adverbs in that an adverb does to a verb, adjective, or other adverbs what an adjective does to a noun. The main function of both adjectives and adverbs is to describe. Adjectives describe nouns; adverbs most commonly describe verbs:

Noun Modifier	**Verb Modifier**
coronary embolism	*usually* found
axillary crutches	*commonly* used
electrical connection	spoke *eloquently*

Adjectives and adverbs can be distinguished by the different types of questions they answer.

Adjectives Answer:	**Adverbs Answer:**
Which one	How
What kind	Where
How many, how much	When
	How many times
	To what extend

- Adverbs tell *how:* "The details in the chart were described *accurately.*"
- Adverbs tell *where:* "The wound bled *locally.*"
- Adverbs tell *when*: "The operation was performed *yesterday.*"
- Adverbs tell *how many times*: "The nurse cleaned the wound *twice.*"
- Adverbs tell *to what extent*: "Insurance costs increased *dramatically.*"

Examples of Adverbs

actually	early	maybe	seriously
afterward	easily	most	somewhere
again	enough	never	soon
ago	entirely	next	still
almost	especially	now	surely
already	everywhere	obviously	there
always	extremely	occasionally	today
anymore	fast	often	together
anywhere	finally	once	tomorrow
apparently	fortunately	orally	too
carefully	generally	perhaps	up
certainly	hard	quite	very
clinically	here	quietly	well
completely	immediately	rarely	where
constantly	just	regularly	yesterday
downward	later	seldom	yet

If you are confused about whether a word is an adjective or an adverb, determine the part of speech that the word describes. If the word modifies a noun, it is an adjective. If the word modifies a verb, it is an adverb. Note, however, that the same word may be either an adjective or an adverb depending on its use in a sentence:

The nurse gave a *daily* report. [*Daily* is an adjective modifying the noun *report.*]

The nurse administered pills *daily.* [*Daily* is an adverb modifying the verb *administered.*]

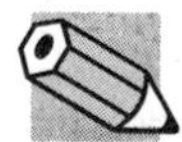

Practice 5-1

Select the adverb in each sentence and identify the question it answers (how, when, where, how many times, or *to what extent):*

1. He is extremely frustrated that he cannot use his dentures. ____________________
2. Periapical areas are checked often. ____________________
3. The flaps were sutured carefully. ____________________
4. The cholesterol levels were checked regularly. ____________________

5. Implants were removed surgically. ____________________

6. The pain lessened after the patient took the medication. ____________________

7. The patient took the medication today. ____________________

8. The patient's record is here on his desk. ____________________

9. The doctor checked the x-rays twice. ____________________

10. Oral hygiene was generally good. ____________________

Adverbs as Modifiers

An adverb is a word that modifies (describes) a verb, verb phrase, adjective, or other adverb. Adverbs that describe verbs are the easiest to identify.

Examples

The patient has recovered *nicely* from the procedure. [*Nicely* modifies the verb *recovered* and answers the question *how.*]

He was casted in the office *yesterday.* [*Yesterday* modifies the verb *casted* and answers the question *when.*]

The medical assistant wrapped the burned area *twice* a day. [*Twice* modifies the verb *wrapped* and answers the questions *how many times.*]

Adverbs can also describe adjectives and other adverbs. Examples of adverbs that perform this function are *very, too, rather, fairly, truly, extremely, unusually, exceptionally, somewhat,* and *especially.* Determining whether the adverb modifies an adjective or adverb depends on how the word is used in a sentence.

Examples

The medical team performed an *especially* safe operation. [*Especially* modifies the adjective safe.]

The incision healed *fairly* rapidly. [*Fairly* modified the adverb *rapidly.*]

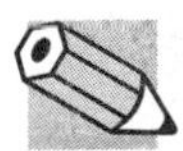

Practice 5-2

Identify the adverb(s) in each sentence and state whether the adverb describes a verb, adjective, or other adverb:

1. This elevator services only surgical patients. ____________________

2. A day in the emergency room passes very quickly. ____________________

3. The M.A. student found the forceps yesterday. ____________________

4. The patient's temperature dropped almost overnight. ____________________

5. The doctor spoke fairly briefly. ________________

6. The hospital generally accepts the H&P prepared by the medical office.
____

7. Cranial nerves II–IV appear grossly intact. ________________

8. We often go to the clinic. ________________

9. The patient tolerated the procedure well. ________________

10. The doctor will probably review the consultation later. ________________

Frequency Adverbs

Specific adverbs exist that describe an amount of time, from full time to no time at all. Some of them are *always, usually, often, sometimes, seldom, rarely,* and *never.*

Examples

I *always* remember.	I *sometimes* remember.
I *usually* remember.	I *rarely* remember.
I *often* remember.	I *never* remember.

The patient *often* reacts to medication.

The report is *usually* filed on Mondays.

We *always* test the blood for HIV.

Degrees of Adverbs to Express Comparison

Adverbs, like adjectives, have three degrees of comparison: positive, comparative, and superlative.

Positive

The positive degree shows no comparison. It is the base form of the adverb.

The progress note was written *clearly.*

Comparative

The comparative degree is used to compare two persons or things that perform the same action. Adverbs ending in *ly* form the comparative by adding the word *more* or *less* immediately before the adverb. Other adverbs form the comparative by adding *er* to the base word.

Examples

The progress note was written *less clearly* than the other one.

James finished the transcription, but Pat did hers *faster.*

Superlative

The superlative degree is used to compare more than two persons or things that perform the same action. To form the superlative degree of adverbs ending in *ly,* add *most* or *least* immediately before the adverb. Other adverbs are also formed by adding *est* to the base form.

Examples

The final progress note was written *least clearly* of all.

The nurse scored the *highest* in the class.

The hospital admitted patients *most cordially.*

Other Comparisons

Some verbs do not form their comparative and superlative degrees according to the rules stated in the previous paragraphs. They are irregular. For example:

Positive	*little*	Dr. Mary Ann cares *little* about covering the emergency room.
Comparative	*less*	Dr. Bill is *less* likely than she to cover the emergency room.
Positive	*least*	Of all the physicians, Dr. Joseph is the *least* likely to cover the emergency room.

Other common irregular adverbs are:

Positive	***Comparative***	***Superlative***
badly	worse	worst
well	better	best
far	farther	farthest
much	more	most

When using the words *more* or *most,* do not make the mistake of also adding the suffix *er* or *est* to adverbs.

Incorrect	Bill worked *more harder* than expected.
Correct	Bill worked *harder* than expected.
Incorrect	We arrived *more earlier* than John.
Correct	We arrived *earlier* than John.

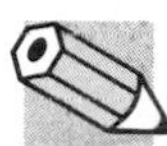

Practice 5-3

Select the correct word in the parentheses:

1. Oral medications are (more, most) acceptable than intramuscular medications.

2. Kelly is (less, least) confident than I am.

3. Of the two choices, the surgical procedure is (more expensive, the most expensive).

4. Doctors train (longer, more longer, most longest) than nurses do to care for the sick.

5. The OR is (busy, busier, most busy) than the ER.

6. Certified mail is the (good, better, best) way to send documents at the post office.

7. Respirators are (scarcist, more scarce) in poorer countries.

8. Telecommunication such as a fax machine and computer-to-computer e-mail is the (fast, faster, fastest) method of communication.

9. More medical supplies are (available, more available, most available) on the Internet.

10. The patient felt badly before, but feels even (badder, worse, worst) now.

Changing Adjectives into Adverbs

Medical words can be expressed as adjectives and adverbs.

Examples

The *medical* prognosis for that patient is serious. (Adjective)

The *prognosis* for that patient is *medically* serious. (Adverb)

1. Simply, add *ly* to the adjective: clinical, clinical*ly*; medical, medical*ly*; physical, physical*ly*; progressive, progressive*ly*; anterior, anterior*ly*; posterior, posterior*ly*; pathological, pathological*ly*.
2. Adjectives that end in *y* preceded by a consonant are made into adverbs by changing the *y* to *i* and adding *ly*: easy, eas*ily*; happy, happ*ily*.
3. Adjectives ending in *le* are made into adverbs by changing the ending to *ly*: probable, probab*ly*; acceptable, acceptab*ly*; justifiable, justifiab*ly*.
4. Adjectives ending in *ll* are made into adverbs by adding *y*: full, full*y*; dull, dull*y*.
5. Adjectives ending in *ic* are usually made into adverbs by adding *ally*: historic, histori*cally*; diagnostic, diagnosti*cally*.
6. Some adverbs have special spellings: tru*ly* publicl*y* whol*ly*

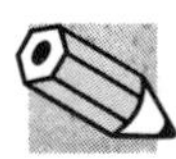

Practice 5-4

Change the following words into adverbs:

1. safe ____________________
2. successful ____________________
3. oral ____________________
4. continual ____________________
5. painful ____________________
6. heavy ____________________
7. spontaneous ____________________
8. specific ____________________
9. basic ____________________
10. frantic ____________________

Negative Adverbs

A negative, the oppositive of affirmative, is a word that expresses a denial or a refusal. A negative contradicts what is said.

John lives in Boston. [affirmative]

John does not live in Boston. [negative]

Regular negative adverbs are *no, not, never, no one, nobody, nothing, nowhere, none, hardly, rarely, barely, scarcely*, and *seldom*. Be aware that the word *no* is also a negative *adjective*. Words like *nobody, nowhere, nothing,* and *no one* are negative *pronouns*. The prefixes *dis-, in-, non-,* and *un-* are also indicators of negatives.

Examples

She *never* goes to the doctor. [Adverb regular]

The treatment room has *no* surgical tape. [adjective]

Nobody can tell me the information I want. [pronoun]

Nothing should stand in the way of improving your health. [pronoun]

I did *not* attend the meeting. [adverb]

*Un*pack the medical supplies that just arrived. [prefix]

The doctor *dis*charged the patient before the weekend. [prefix]

Not as a Contraction

The adverb *not* is often joined to verbs to create a new word. The new word is called a contraction. To form a contraction, an apostrophe (') replaces the letter *o* in the word *not (n't)*. Because the abbreviated form of *not* is implied in the contraction, it is considered a negative word.

Examples

are not	*aren't*	cannot	*can't*	could not	*couldn't*
				would not	*wouldn't*
did not	*didn't*	does not	*doesn't*	do not	*don't*
has not	*hasn't*	have not	*haven't*	had not	*hadn't*
is not	*isn't*	must not	*mustn't*	should not	*shouldn't*
was not	*wasn't*	were not	*weren't*	will not	*won't*

Many people use the contraction *ain't* in their speech. This word is unacceptable in the English language and should not be used, especially in formal writing. Actually, contractions in general are usually avoided in formal writing.

Double Negatives

Another grammatical error that should be avoided is the use of two negatives in a sentence. In such a case, the second negative cancels the first negative and turns the whole sentence into an affirmative. An example is the sentence, "I haven't no money." If you do not have have *no* money, it means you have some money.

Incorrect	The policy *didn't* offer *no* deductible.
Correct	The policy offered *no* deductible.
	The policy didn't offer *any* deductible.
Incorrect	The medical assistants *didn't* have *no* money.
Correct	The medical assistants have *no* money.
	The medical assistants *didn't* have *any* money.

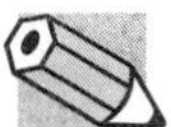

Practice 5-5

Correct these double-negative sentences:

1. I don't hardly ever drink six to eight glasses of water a day. ___________________
2. The insurance company can't pay none of its bills. ___________________
3. They didn't expect no injuries. ___________________
4. The nurse won't have no difficulty telling the patients. ___________________
5. There ain't no positions at this time. ___________________
6. The DRGs used by Medicare hasn't had no effect on billing. ___________________
7. The medication couldn't scarcely work after two hours. ___________________
8. Changes in schedule didn't make nobody happy. ___________________
9. I didn't do nothing wrong. ___________________
10. She doesn't want none of my help. ___________________

Placement of Adverbs

If adverbs and adjectives are not placed near the words they describe, they can provide the reader with a good laugh. For example, the sentence, "She promised him that she would marry him frequently," should read, "She frequently promised him that she would marry him." Which is the intended meaning; how many times did she promise to marry him, or how many times did she actually marry him?

Adverbs that modify adjectives or adverbs are placed immediately before the words they describe:

Awkward	Luke said that he was going to the office emphatically.
Better	Luke emphatically said that he was going to the office.

Adverbs that modify verbs can be placed in many positions in a sentence:

The doctor listened *intently* to the patient's symptoms.

The doctor listened to the patient's symptoms *intently*.

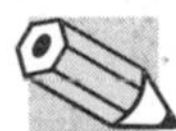

Practice 5-6

Place the adverb from the first column in its best position in the sentence:

1. always	Sue has a yearly physical.
2. ever	Have you had an operation on your gallbladder?
3. seldom	The office opens earlier than 9 a.m.
4. usually	Medical assistants work very hard.
5. probably	For this reason, nurses need help.
6. highly	Students are acclaimed when they qualify for medical school.
7. immediately	Get her to the operating room.
8. especially	On busy days, the medial assistant works later.
9. courageously	The patient signed a health care proxy.
10. rarely	Doctors make mistakes in diagnosing obvious diseases.

Troublesome Adverbs

The following words are often confused.

awhile:	The doctor paused *awhile* during the difficult surgery. [adverb]	*a + while*:	There was silence in the ER for *a while*. [noun]
well:	The patient feels *well*. [adverb]	*good*:	The woman had a *good* doctor. [noun]
really:	I was *really* expecting a bonus. [adverb]	*real*:	The patient had a *real* greenstick fracture. [adjective]
surely:	You can *surely* count on me for help when you are ill. [adverb]	*sure*:	The diagnosis is a *sure* thing. [adjective]

Medical Spelling

Become familiar with the spelling of the following words:

abnormally — accurately

absolutely — analysis

apparently	nutritionally
axillary	occasionally
carefully	orally
chronically	particularly
clinically	physically
confidentially	possibly
currently	posteriorly
developmentally	potentially
dorsally	primarily
emotionally	radically
immediately	relatively
initially	significantly
insufficiently	specifically
intramuscularly	temporarily
intravenously	timely
involuntarily	tomorrow
laterally	ventrally
locally	yesterday

Adverbs Study Summary

Definition	A word that describes a verb, adjective, or other adverb.	The operation was *successfully* completed.
Question answered	*How? where? when? how many times? to what extent?*	Treatments have to be administered *often*. (how many times) The answer may be found *here*. (where)
Placement	Immediately near adjective, anywhere with adverb.	What is needed are *extremely* safe guidelines.
Comparative and superlative		
One syllable	Add *er, est*: fast, faster, fastest.	This method is *faster* than the other one.
Two syllables Three syllables	Add *more, most*: more impatient, most impatient	She replied most *impatiently*.
Irregular	*Well, better, best* *Badly, worst, worst*	This is the *worst* I have ever felt.
Avoid double comparatives	Do not use *er, est* endings with more and most: more easy, *not* more easier, most easy, *not* most easiest.	Avoid at all cost.

Avoid double negatives	Do not use two negatives in a sentence for example: *not, rarely, seldom, hardly, scarcely, barely.*	Avoid at all cost.

Skills Review

Add to the sentence the type of adverb that is described in the parentheses:

1. The patient ate his meal. (adverb telling how) ____________________
2. The patient ate his meal. (adverb telling where) ____________________
3. A low-fat diet was ordered. (adverb telling when) ____________________
4. The patient had physical therapy. (adverb telling how many times) ____________________
5. The patient ambulated to the door and back. (how) ____________________
6. The pain increased. (how) ____________________
7. The cancer spread. (to what extent) ____________________
8. Phil spoke to his mother. (how) ____________________
9. The man seemed apprehensive. (to what extent) ____________________
10. The elevator stopped. (where) ____________________

Identify the modifiers and state whether they are adverbs or adjectives:

1. The patient required radical surgery. ____________________
2. A highly complex problem existed. ____________________
3. Christopher felt apprehensive going to the hospital. ____________________
4. They finally finished their work. ____________________
5. The femur is the largest bone in the body. ____________________
6. A local anesthetic was used. ____________________
7. Xylocaine was used locally. ____________________
8. The chronic pain was treated with morphine. ____________________
9. The incision was made laterally ____________________
10. The medication was given orally. ____________________

Give the comparative and superlative forms of these adverbs:

1. fast ______________ ______________
2. badly ______________ ______________
3. lovingly ______________ ______________
4. poor ______________ ______________
5. carefully ______________ ______________
6. late ______________ ______________
7. little ______________ ______________
8. dangerously ______________ ______________
9. dreary ______________ ______________
10. rich ______________ ______________

Rewrite these sentences, if necessary.

1. The doctor won't order no laxative.

   ____

2. Don't change no facts on the medical record.

   ____

3. The patient's temperature hasn't hardly risen all day.

   ____

4. The doctor doesn't need none of the information until tomorrow.

   ____

5. The operation wasn't never cancelled.

   ____

6. Nothing couldn't hardly stop the bleeding.

   ____

7. The patient never runs no temperature.

____

8. Medication didn't give the patient no reaction.

____

9. We don't usually do no surgeries in the evening.

____

10. This sphygmomanometer won't never be useful again.

____

Circle the correct word within the parentheses:

1. After taking her pills, the patient felt (good, well).
2. The nurse hadn't told (anybody, nobody) about the patient.
3. OSHA standards protect employees who may be (occupational, occupationally) exposed to infectious material.
4. We heard (nothing, anything) about the doctor's report.
5. The patients had (no, nothing) history of contagious diseases.
6. Edward wasn't (ever, never) in the emergency room.
7. The victim couldn't (hardly, ever) survive the accident.
8. There is exposure to blood or other (potential, potentially) infectious material.
9. The answer to the problem was (probably, probable) easy to solve.
10. Remove all protective clothing (immediate, immediately) upon leaving the work area.

Circle the correctly spelled word in each line:

1. chronicaly	kronically	chroncally	chronically
2. portnetally	potentiantlly	potentially	protentially
3. signifcanntly	signifikantly	significantly	sigfically
4. intervenously	intrevenously	intervously	intravenously

5. primarely	primarily	premarily	primerily
6. developementally	deveolpmentally	developmentally	defelopmentally
7. imediatelly	immediately	imediately	immedeately
8. confidentally	confedintialy	confidentilly	confidentially
9. dorsally	dorsilly	dorsaly	dorsully
10. latirally	laterally	latarally	lateraly

Write a different adverb in each circle to modify the verb and an adjective to modify the noun. Use words that apply to a medical situation.

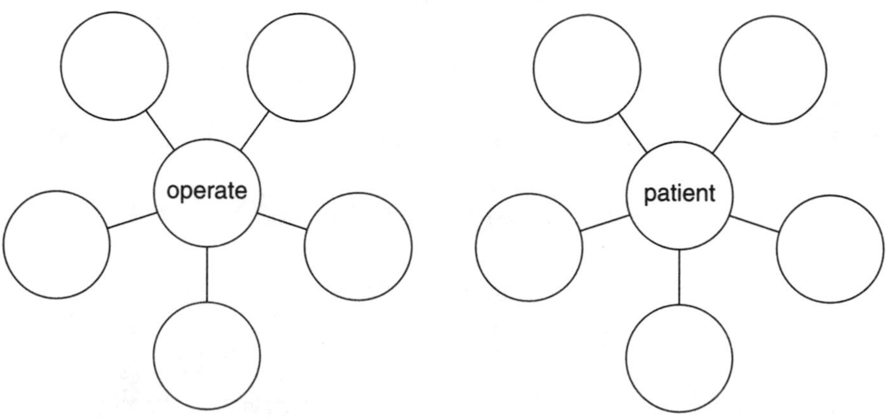

Write five sentences using adverbs. Circle the adverb and underline the verb, adjective, or adverb it describes. Use words that apply in a medical situation.

1. ______________________________
2. ______________________________
3. ______________________________
4. ______________________________
5. ______________________________

Translate medical abbreviations using a medical dictionary or appendix.

1. KUB ______________
2. LE ______________
3. LP ______________

4. mEq ____________________

5. LUQ ____________________

6. MI ____________________

7. mg ____________________

8. NKA ____________________

9. NPO ____________________

10. NSAID ____________________

Chapter 6

Prepositions and Conjunctions

Objectives

Upon completion of this chapter, the student should be able to:

- recognize prepositions, compound prepositions, and prepositional phrases
- use prepositional phrases as modifiers
- understand problematic prepositions
- recognize coordinating, correlative, and subordinating conjunctions
- spell various medical terms
- translate various medical abbreviations

Prepositions

A preposition shows how a noun or pronoun is related to another word or group of words in a sentence. It is a connective word that joins a noun or pronoun to the rest of the sentence. Prepositions are used very often in speaking and writing.

Examples

Sociology is the study *of* the origins *of* society.

Anatomy is the science *of* the structure *of* the body and the relationship *of* its parts.

"Physio-" refers *to* nature. Physiology is the study *of* the functions and activities *of* the living body.

Radiopaque means impenetrable *to* x-rays. X-rays do not go *through* metals.

Calcium causes bones *to* be radiopaque. Calcification is when deposits *of* calcium harden organic tissues.

Dr. Jack and Dr. Jill went *up* the hall *to* fetch a liter *of* I.V. fluid.

Dr. Jack fell *down* the hall and broke his arm. Dr. Jill came tumbling *after* him.

The words in italics, the prepositions, show the relationship to the nouns and pronouns in the sentences.

Some prepositions help to show location or place: *between, below, near, on, against, in, away,* and *through.*

Examples

Lateral is situated *away* from the midline of the body.

Intercostal is *between* the ribs.

Subcostal means *below* a rib.

Decline means *to* go down *to* something lower.

Dorsal means toward or situated *on* the back side.

The medical report is *on* the table.

In the anatomical position, the body is facing forward *with* the arms *at* the sides and the palms *toward* the front.

A few prepositions show a relationship of time: *before, during, since,* and *until.*

Examples

Before performing the examination, wash your hands carefully.

The intern fell asleep *during* the lecture.

I can't pay my medical loans *until* I get a job.

During the delivery of the Rh-negative baby, some of the baby's blood cells containing antigens may escape *into* the mother's bloodstream.

Other prepositions show different kinds of relationships between a noun or pronoun and another word: *about, among, by, for, from, like, of, to,* and *with.*

Examples

Rh immune globulin is given *to* the mother *to* help prevent the antigen-antibody reaction.

Antibiotic inhibits the growth *of* microorganisms.

Biopsy is the examination *of* tissue *from* the body.

The biopsy was taken *from* the lymph node.

A professional relationship exists *among* doctors and health care professionals.

Some prepositions indicate direction: around, beside, under, through, across, over, toward, and to.

Examples

The sterile drape was placed *over* the Mayo stand.

The cast is molded *around* the contours of the body.

Place the tourniquet *around* the arm three or four inches *above* the venipuncture site.

The physical therapist put the patient *through* range of motion exercises.

Common Prepositions		
about	between	on/onto
above	beyond	out/outside
across	by	over
after	concerning	past
against	despite	round
along	down	regarding
amid	during	since
among	except	through, throughout
around	for	till
as	from	to, toward
at	in/into	under, underneath
before	inside/outside	until
behind	like	unto
below	near	up/upon
beneath	of	with/without/within
beside/besides	off	

Compound Prepositions

Compound prepositions are two or three words that are used so frequently together that they function like one-word prepositions.

Commonly Used Compound Prepositions		
according to	in addition to	in terms of
along with	in back of	in support of
apart from	in connection with	next to
as for	in contrast to	on account of
as regards	in defense of	on behalf of
as to	in front of	out of
aside from	in place of	together with
because of	in reference to	with reference to
by way of	in regard to	with regard to
contrary to	in spite of	with respect to
due to	instead of	

Prepositional Phrase

A prepositional phrase begins with a preposition and ends with a noun or pronoun that is its object.

Examples

by next Wednesday	under the fascia
through the bloodstream	for the patient
at work	regarding the long-term prognosis

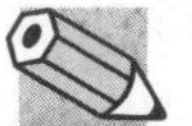

Practice 6-1

Underline the prepositional phrases:

1. By next Thursday, our accounts should be balanced.
2. Throughout the exam, Mrs. Griffs was very cooperative and without pain.
3. The medical assistant's instructions to the patient about the diet should be on the paper.
4. The liver removes bilirubin from the blood.
5. A bland diet is restricted in flavor and used for patients with gastrointestinal problems.
6. Vitamin K aids in the clotting of blood and is responsible for the production of prothrombin.
7. Vitamin D aids in the building of bones and the body's use of calcium and phosphorus.
8. A hernia of the diaphragm is treated surgically by herniorrhaphy.
9. The normal pulse rate for toddlers and very young children is 80 to 100 pulsations per minute.
10. The Trendelenburg position is used in cases of shock and in some abdominal surgery.

A word of caution regarding compound prepositions: Avoid using two or three words when a single word will suffice.

Examples

Compound	Place the patient's medication *next to* the file.
Singular	Place the patient's medication *beside* the file.
Compound	Medical supplies are kept *inside of* the cabinet
Singular	Medical supplies are kept *in* the cabinet.
Compound	Rose is doing well *in spite of* her sickness.
Singular	Rose is doing well *despite* her sickness.
Compound	Rubber gloves are placed *down under* the shelf.
Singular	Rubber gloves are placed *under* the shelf.

Compound	Medical assistants' uniforms are made *out of* synthetic materials.
Singular	Medical assistants' uniforms are made *of* synthetic materials.

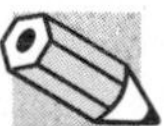

Practice 6-2

Underline the compound preposition and its object:

1. According to the physician's treatment plan, the patient is to undergo chemotherapy.
2. Because of the metastasis of the cancer, the surgeons decided to close the incision.
3. Dr. Villes spoke in support of the consultation.
4. On behalf of my staff, I wish to thank the employees for their dedicated service.
5. With respect to the involved personnel, this has been a team effort.

Prepositional Noun/Pronoun Modifiers

A preposition and the accompanying word or words that form the prepositional phrase are often used to modify a noun or pronoun. Such phrases are usually found in one of two positions: after the word being modified or after a linking verb.

Examples

An *assistant* to the doctor made the travel arrangements to the conference.

The purpose of splinting prevents *motion* of the injured part.

The medical report *is* on the table.

He *is* in the waiting room.

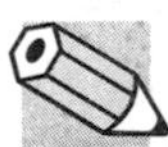

Practice 6-3

Circle the noun and underline the prepositional phrase modifying it:

1. An insurance company charges a premium for its coverage.
2. A patient with emphysema uses the Fowler's position.
3. The autoclave in the treatment room is working.
4. All employees in the medical office must observe asepsis.
5. Hypertension is a major contributor to heart attacks.

Prepositional Verb Modifiers

Prepositional phrases can also modify verbs and answer the questions *how? when? where?* and *to what extent*?

Examples

The postural drainage is done *by cupping and clapping the hands over the patients shoulder blades.* [how? where?]

The tricuspid valve is located *in the heart.* [where?]

The medication must be taken *with meals.* [when?]

The surgeon dictates the surgical procedure *in great detail.* [to what extent?]

Prepositional phrases that modify verbs can occupy different positions in the sentence, thus enabling the writer to emphasize different points.

Examples

At last, the patient agreed to undergo treatment.

The patient agreed *at last* to undergo treatment.

The patient agreed to undergo treatment *at last.*

Good writing focuses on the reader rather than the writer. Starting a sentence with the word *I* can easily be avoided by beginning the sentence with a prepositional phrase instead.

Examples

On Friday, I spoke to the x-ray technician.

In spite of the work involved, I want to write the article for the medical journal.

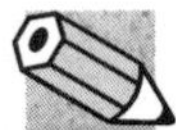

Practice 6-4

Circle the modified verb and underline the prepositional phrase:

1. Urinary output is recorded by measuring the amount voided.
2. Repression occurs when painful thoughts are forced into the unconscious.
3. Tissues that are removed in surgery are sent to pathology.
4. Illness is denied through defense mechanisms.
5. Viruses live within other cells and can only be seen by electron microscopes.

Circle all of the prepositions *in this paragraph:*

"I will follow that system of regimen which, according to my ability and judgment, I consider for the benefit of my patients, and abstain from whatever is deleterious and mischievous. I will give no deadly medicine to anyone if asked, nor suggest any such counsel; and in like manner I will not give to a woman a pessary to produce abortion. With purity and with holiness I will pass my life and practice my art. I will not cut persons laboring under the stone, but will leave this to be done by men who are practitioners of the work. Into whatever houses I enter, I will go into them for the benefit of the sick, and I will abstain from every voluntary act of mischief and corruption; and, further, from the seduction of females or males, of freemen and slaves. Whatever, in connection with my professional practice, or not in connection with it, I see or hear, in the life of men, which ought not to be spoken of abroad, I will not divulge, as reckoning that all such should be kept secret." (Taken from the Hippocratic Oath)

Problematic Prepositions

Prepositions that often cause difficulty in writing are *between* and *among*, and *beside* and *besides*. *Between* refers to two people, things, or groups and *among* refers to more than two:

> Information *between* a patient and a physician is highly confidential.
>
> *Among* all the students in the class, she was the one who worked in the OR.

Beside means "next to" and besides means "in addition to" or "except":

> The oxygen tank is *beside* the bed.
>
> There is another insurance company *besides* that HMO that offers the benefits.

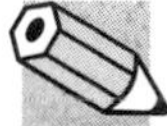

Practice 6-5

Identify the correct word within parentheses:

1. (Beside, Besides) radiation, the patient must also have chemotherapy.
2. This information is shared (among, between) the doctor and the patient.
3. The medication was placed (beside, besides) the glass of water.
4. The pain medication is usually taken (among, between) the hours of five and seven o'clock.
5. The hospital is located (beside, besides) the university structure.
6. Hospital physicians are (among, between) the personnel who attended the meeting.
7. Put the chair (beside, besides) the patient's bed.
8. Corridors (between, among) the first and second floor must be locked.
9. Can anyone (beside, besides) Dr. Villes perform the operation?
10. One person stood out (between, among) the crowd.

Other prepositions that often are misused are *to, different from, in,* and *into.* The problem with the preposition *to* is that it sounds like the words *two* and *too. To* is a preposition meaning toward something, *two* is a number and a noun, and *too* is an adverb meaning "also":

John went *to* the science lab.

Two opinions are needed by the insurance company.

I'd like more medical information, *too*.

Confusion exists about the use of the preposition *from* after the word *different*. The preferred expression is *different from* rather than *different than*.

Use *different from* when it means the same as "differs from something else":

The recommendation was *different from* ours.

Use *different than* with the comparative degree of adjectives and adverbs:

Mr. Jones's training was *different than* Mr. Smith's.

The preposition *in* refers to a location or movement within an area:

The file is *in* Dr. Villes's office.

The preposition *into* means "entry, introduction, insertion, superposition, or inclusion":

The doctor and lawyer entered *into* a mutual agreement, and then the patient came *into* the conference room.

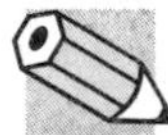

Practice 6-6

Identify the correct word to be used from within the parentheses:

1. Nurses' uniforms are (different than, different from) years ago.
2. The supervisor wanted the nurse to look (in, into) the causes of the injury.
3. At times, doctors work (to, too, two) shifts at a time.
4. Nurses often work overtime (to, too, two).
5. A heart operation is very (different than, different from) a lung operation.
6. Medical personnel entered (in, into) a discussion about cancer treatment.
7. The expectant father paced (into, in) the delivery room.
8. The hospital was accredited for (two, to, too) additional years.
9. Isopropyl alcohol is used to clean the surface of the skin, (to, too, two).
10. Put the specimen (in, into) the container.

Prepositions at the End of a Sentence

Many English instructors maintain that a sentence ending with a preposition is weak. However, it is an acceptable practice to do so in certain situations:

When the preposition is part of the previous verb.

Examples

I am sending you some reports to look *at*. Read them *through*.

The medical team can be counted *on*.

If the end preposition emphasizes a strong point.

Examples

The side effects were too much to contend *with*.

Where did the cancer metastasize *from*?

In formal writing, it is best to try to place the preposition anywhere but at the end or to rewrite (but without being awkward).

Examples

Medicare is for patients age 65 years of age or *over*.

Medicare is for patients *over* 65 years of age.

Death and dying is a difficult subject *about* which to talk.

The subject of death and dying is difficult to talk *about*.

Examples

Chris is the person I work *with*. I work *with* Chris.

What is the book *about*? The book is *about* what?

Where is this medication shipped *to*? Where is the medication shipped?

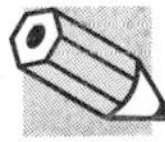

Practice 6-7

Rearrange the preposition within the sentence or otherwise revise for clarity:

1. Who am I going to vote *for*? ____________________
2. These symptoms are something I never heard *of*. ____________________
3. Cathy feels it necessary to drain the water *off*. ____________________
4. I changed the dressing before and *after* physical therapy. ____________________
5. The patient's scream from the emergency room was heard *throughout*. ____________________
6. You're the third patient I've attended *to*. ____________________
7. Never keep the medicines *underneath*. ____________________
8. Later this evening, I hope to look *around*. ____________________

9. What are you in the hospital *for*? ____________________

10. The anesthesiologist put the patient *under*? ____________________

Conjunctions

A conjunction is another part of speech that joins words or parts of sentences. There are three types: coordinating, correlative, and subordinating.

Coordinating Conjunctions

The coordinating conjunctions *and, but, or,* and *yet* are used to join two single words or groups of words of the same kind or of equal construction.

Examples

Dr. Hebert *and* Dr. Balin prepared for surgery. [The conjunction *and* joins two proper nouns, *Dr. Hebert* and *Dr. Balin,* to form a compound subject.]

Ask Kate *or* Jane to cover the main desk. [The word *or* connects or joins the two indirect objects, *Kate* and *Jane.*]

His speech was short *but* effective. [*But* connects the equal construction of the two predicate adjectives, *short* and *effective.*]

She said she'd be late, *yet* she arrived on time. [*Yet* connects the group of words relating the similar constructions, *she'd be late* and *she arrived on time.*]

Correlative Conjunction

Correlative conjunctions consist of two elements used as pairs to connect parallel structures.

both . . . and	*Both* the doctor *and* the nurse were present.
not only . . . but also	The machine *not only* copies materials *but also* sorts.
either . . . or	*Either* I *or* my assistant will be in the ER.
whether . . . or	I'm going *whether* you are *or* you're not.
neither . . . nor	*Neither* the doctor *nor* the nurse could contain the patient on the stretcher.

Subordinating Conjunction

The subordinating conjunction begins an adverb clause and joins the clause to the sentence. This type of conjunction is covered in detail in Chapter 7 on clauses and phrases.

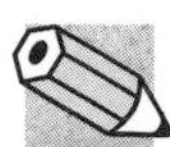

Practice 6-8

Identify the conjunction and state whether it is coordinating or correlative:

1. Give Valerie or Christopher a call at the hospital. ____________________

2. Both chemotherapy and radiation are needed for this type of cancer. ________________

3. The medical assistants studied long and hard. ________________

4. The incision was not only painful but also inflamed. ________________

5. Either Dr. Villes or Dr. Archie will be on call this weekend. ________________

6. Runny nose and general malaise are symptoms of a cold. ________________

7. He broke his lower back and femur in the accident. ________________

8. You can either make a dental appointment now or later. ________________

9. The patient may eat and drink after the blood is drawn. ________________

10. Either set the fracture now or bring the patient for a CT scan. ________________

Medical Spelling

Become familiar with the spelling of the following words:

antiemetic
antihistamines
asepsis
asphyxia
autoclave
bilirubin
cyanotic
deficiency
diaphoresis
diaphragm
electrode
eliminated
fascia
flatulence
Fowler's position
fumigation
hazardous
hypertension
isopropyl
lithotomy
manipulation
metastasis
nausea
palpitation
percussion
postprandial
prothrombin
pruritus
regime
regimen
sanitization
semi-Fowler's
specimen
sterilization
syncope
technique
Trendelenburg
urticaria
vertigo
viruses

Prepositions and Conjunctions Study Summary

Preposition Shows how a noun/pronoun is related to another word or group of words in a sentence; a connective word that joins a noun/pronoun to the rest of the sentence: "The letter continues *on* the next page."

Compound prepositions	Two to three words that function like one preposition.	I'm calling *in regard to* the package I received *by way of* Federal Express.
Prepositional phrases	Begins with a preposition and ends with a noun or pronoun that is its object.	The procedure took place *in the operating room.*
Prepositional modifiers:		
Noun/pronoun	Found after the word modified or after a linking verb.	The reason *for the meeting* is obvious. The reports are filed *under the letter S.*
Verb modifiers	Modifies a verb and answers *how? when? where? and to what extend?*	The answer is found *in the last chapter.* (where) The medication is taken *before going to bed.* (when)
Problematic prepositions	Between—refers to two.	This information is just *between* us.
	Among—refers to more than two.	Patience is listed *among* the qualities.
	Beside—next to.	Stand *beside* me during the announcement.
	Besides—in addition to.	*Besides* the book there is a map.
	To—the preposition.	Go *to* the OR STAT!
	Two—the number.	*Two* problems exist in the report.
	Too—also.	I'm going, *too.*
	Different from is the preferred expression over different than.	This treatment is different *from* the last one.
Prepositions at the end of a sentence	An acceptable practice: When preposition is part of a previous verb. Emphasizes a strong point Try to avoid it at the end in formal writing.	This is one thing you have to attend *to.*

Conjunction Joins words or parts of sentences

Coordinating Joins two single words or groups of words of the same kind or equal construction: *and, but, yet.* "Vitamin D is found in liver, butter, *and* green vegetables." "The wound is healing, *yet* it still needs to be covered."

Correlative Pairs of words used to connect parallel structures:

both . . . and: "*Both* Ben *and* his wife are sick."

not only . . . but also: "The doctor is *not only* a surgeon *but also* an instructor."

either . . . or: "*Either* the patient comes in today *or* sometime next week."

whether . . . or: "*Whether* the scrubs are green *or* yellow is up to you."

neither . . . nor: "*Neither* the x-ray *nor* other tests revealed any problem."

Subordinating Begins an adverb clause and joins it to the sentence: "*Before* she left the doctor's office, she paid her copayment."

Skills Review

Circle the prepositions in the following paragraph:

John Doe is a 23-year old male suffering from back pain and memory loss as a result of injuries sustained in a car accident three months ago. At that time, the patient was the driver of an automobile traveling across Main to State Street. Another vehicle hit Mr. Doe's car on the front passenger's side before coming to a halt. Complaining of pain with any movement of his neck, John was transported by ambulance to the emergency department of Wells Medical Center. X-rays of the cervical spine revealed an injury affecting his neck and back. He was placed on a high dose of anti-inflammatory medication and muscle relaxants, and provided with a cervical collar. Because of the accident, John Doe has been unable to work since the motor vehicle accident in question.

Write the correct preposition in the blanks:

1. The study ________________ diseases ________________ the elderly is called geriatrics.
2. Proximal is ________________ the point of attachment.
3. An oncologist is concerned ________________ cancer.
4. Ventral and anterior pertain ________________ the front of the body.
5. The patient lost much blood ________________ the delivery of her child.
6. Everyone ________________ the technicians were in the room.
7. A tour was given ________________ the hospital
8. Turn right ________________ the elevator and take your first left.
9. ________________ the intercom, Dr. Ville was paged three times.
10. Surgeries were running ________________ schedule.

Supply a coordinating or correlative conjunction:

1. ________________ apples ________________ oranges have healthy nutritional value.
2. Mary will not attend the meeting, ________________ Brad will.
3. The medical assistant looked for the report ________________ could not find it.
4. Oh, but doctors also need knowledge, experience, ________________ compassion.
5. ________________ scholarships ________________ grants are available for research.
6. The responsibility belongs ________________ to you ________________ and your assistant.
7. Make sure the patient is conscious enough to eat ________________ swallow.
8. Explain the procedure ________________ follow-up treatment.
9. ________________ we obtain the blood test ________________ we give glucose in the form of orange juice.
10. Each person may experience diabetes in his or her own unique way ________________ pattern.

Circle the correctly spelled word in each line:

1. Trendelanburg	Trendilenburg	Trendelenburg	Trendelonburg
2. hypirtension	hipertension	hypertision	hypertension
3. virus'	viruss	viruses	virusas
4. technikue	tehneque	tecknique	technique
5. urticaria	urtkaria	urtecaria	urtocaria
6. defencency	deficiency	dificiency	deficeincy
7. metaztazis	metatsasis	matastasis	metastasis
8. facia	fascia	faccsia	fassia
9. cianotic	cyantoic	cyanotic	ciaanotyc
10. diaphigm	diafragm	diaphragm	diephragm

Skills Review on the Parts of Speech

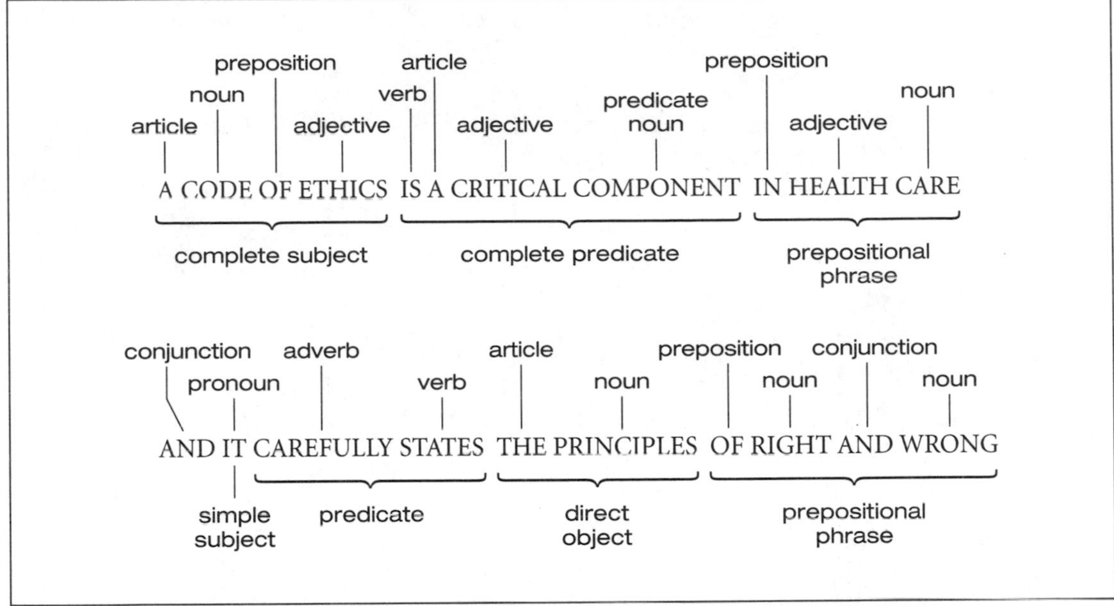

Review of Parts of Speech and Usage

Write the corresponding part of speech from the list below above each italicized word in the sentences.

noun	adverb	article	adjective
pronoun	preposition	conjunction	verb

1. *Somebody* in the family has to learn how to deal with a potential diabetic emergency.
2. The tickler file is a *reminder* file.
3. Respiration is the process *of* breathing.
4. Patients facing death *pass* through many emotional and psychological stages.
5. Glucose tolerance testing is contraindicated for patients with recent surgery *or* myocardial infarctions.
6. Minerals are calcium, phosphorus, iodine, iron, copper, *and* potassium.
7. The man was having *severe* chest pain during the procedure.
8. *The* Patient's Bill of Rights is a set of laws that helps protect patients.
9. OSHA suggests safety *measures* that must be taken to prevent or limit the spread of germs.
10. Limiting the use of antibiotics is crucial for the prevention of bacterial growth *and* resistance.

11. The lungs were *very* congested.

12. The test for BUN is used as a gross index of glomerular *function* and the production and excretion of urea.

13. A *medical* doctor who treats mental illness is a psychiatrist.

14. PSA is not a definitive test for prostate *cancer* .

15. The medical assistant makes the *patients'* appointments.

Write the part of speech above each word in the sentence:

1. Document telephone calls in a medical office.

2. Ask the patient which arm he or she prefers for the phlebotomy.

3. Schedule the ultrasound for Wednesday.

4. An artery is a vessel that carries blood to the heart.

5. Check the prescription and order at the pharmacy.

Translate medical abbreviations using a medical dictionary or appendix.

1. OOB ____________________

2. O.S. ____________________

3. OR ____________________

4. o.u. ____________________

5. ORIF ____________________

6. p.c. ____________________

7. PERRLA ____________________

8. p.o. ____________________

9. p.r.n. ____________________

10. PTT ____________________

Section Two

Phrases, Clauses, Sentences, and Paragraphs

Chapter 7

Phrases and Clauses

Objectives *Upon completion of this chapter, students should be able to:*

- understand how phrases function within the structure of a sentence
- recognize various types of phrases
- understand how clauses function within the structure of a sentence
- recognize various types of dependent clauses
- spell various medical terms
- translate various medical abbreviations

The previous six chapters explained how words are used as single parts of speech. This chapter shows how groups of words function as parts of a sentence.

Phrases

A phrase is a group of words without a subject or a predicate.

Examples

toward the patient's face *on the operating table*

in the left kidney *to cure the disease*

Consider these phrases within the context of a sentence:

Subject and Predicate	***Phrase (No Subject or Predicate)***
Urticaria is spreading	*toward the patient's face.*
Calculi were found	*in the left kidney.*
The patient died	*on the operating table.*
Oncologists tried	*to cure the disease.*

Note that the subjects and predicates in these sentences can function independently as complete sentences because they have a subject and a predicate:

Urticaria is spreading.

Calculi were found.

The patient died.

Oncologists tried.

The phrases—*toward the patient's face, in the left kidney, on the operating table,* and *to cure the disease*—however, cannot exist independently because they have no subject or predicate.

Prepositional Phrase

Most phrases in the English language are prepositional phrases. As stated in Chapter 6, a prepositional phrase is a group of words that begins with a preposition and ends with a noun or pronoun that is its object. The phrases, *toward the patient's face, in the left kidney, on the operating table,* and *to cure the disease,* all contain prepositions, along with nouns and their modifiers.

Preposition	***Modifier***	***Object (Noun or Pronoun)***
toward	the patient's	face
in	the left	kidney
on	the operating	table
to	cure	the disease

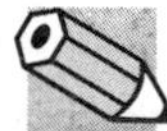

Practice 7-1

Identify the prepositional phrases in the following sentences:

1. Tenderness was noted over the right bicipital tendon.
2. The patient went through lithotripsy.
3. The glomerulus is the filtration unit of the kidney.
4. Nephrectomy is excision of a kidney.
5. The prescription was given over the phone.
6. The patient has cirrhosis of the liver.
7. Cirrhosis is the degeneration of the parenchyma of the liver.
8. The patient presented with hematemesis in the ER.
9. They used an endoscope viewing the inside of the body.
10. Doctors and nurses from the Forms Committee wrote the H&P format.

Prepositional Phrase Used As a Noun

Prepositional phrases may function in the same manner as nouns. Consult Chapter One.

Prepositional Phrase Used As an Adjective

Prepositional phrases can modify words in the same manner as do adjectives or adverbs. An adjective phrase is a prepositional phrase that describes a noun or pronoun. Adjective phrases, like adjectives, answer the questions *which one? what kind?* or *how many?* and occupy different positions in a sentence.

Examples

A patient *in room 210* is scheduled for a cholecystogram. [The prepositional phrase *in room 210* describes the noun *patient* by answering *which one?* Therefore, it is an adjective phrase.]

The procedure *with few side effects* is the best alternative. [*With few side effects* describes the noun *procedure.*]

The pathology report *with tissue results* is due tomorrow. [*With tissue results* describes the noun *report.*]

Prepositional Phrase Used As an Adverb

An adverb phrase is a prepositional phrase that describes a verb, adjective, or another adverb by answers the questions *how? what? when? why? where?* and *to what extent?* Adverb phrases occupy different positions in a sentence.

Examples

Fortunately for the *students,* no additional courses were required. [The phrase *for the students* modifies the adverb *fortunately* and answers the question *why?*

Nurses worked *without a break.* [The phrase *without a break* modifies the verb *worked* and answers the question *how?*]

The operating room is located conveniently near the recovery room. [The phrase *near the recovery room,* modifies the adverb *conveniently* and answers the question *where?*

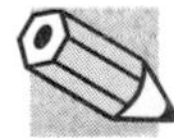

Practice 7-2

Identify the prepositional phrase in each sentence as adjective or adverb:

1. The needle went smoothly into the vein.
2. Surgery is an option for cancer patients.
3. Room 210 is available for a new patient.
4. Unfortunately for the patient, the symptoms indicate glomerulonephritis.
5. Blood in the urine is abnormal.
6. The patient went to physical therapy daily.
7. Polyuria is an indication of diabetes mellitus.
8. Urology is the study of the urinary tract.

9. A nephrectomy was performed reluctantly because of kidney failure.

10. The cystoscopy is scheduled for today.

Verbal Phrases

A verbal is a nonfinite verb—a verb form that does not make a complete sentence—used as a noun, adjective, or adverb. Participles, gerunds, and infinitives are verbals. A verbal phase is a group of words including a verbal and its subject, object, complement, or modifiers that functions as a noun, adjective, or adverb. There are three types of verbal phrases: participial, gerund, and infinitive.

Participial Phrase

A participle is a verb form ending in *ing* (the present participle) or *t, d, ed, en* or other form of the past participle that functions as part of a verbal phrase called a *participial phrase.* A participial phrase usually functions as an *adjective.*

Examples

The patient, *feeling ill,* took the prescribed medicine. [The participial phrase, *feeling ill,* modifies the noun patient. *Feeling* is the present participle of the verb *feel.*]

The culture *taken from the wound,* tested positive for streptococci. [The participial phrase, *taken from the wound,* modifies the noun *culture.*

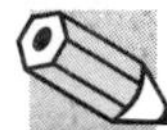

Practice 7-3

Identify the participial phrase in each sentence:

1. The sterilized instruments wrapped with tape were removed from the autoclave.

2. The patient's voice, weakened from laryngitis, was barely heard.

3. Having read the report, she noticed the anomaly.

4. The medical assistant, working the night shift, filled the prescriptions.

5. Trying to keep the information confidential, Dr. Moore was careful with his words.

6. Instructors, understanding their role as mentors, work hard to teach positive values.

7. Physicians, experiencing the pressure of the HMO, need to take control.

8. The sphygmomanometer mounted on the wall is found in the examination room.

9. Immunizations, given throughout childhood, are recommended by the Public Health Department.

10. Volunteers, retired from careers, perform valuable services in hospitals.

Gerund Phrase

A gerund is a verb form ending in *ing* that is used in any way that a noun may be used: as a subject, object, object of a preposition, or predicate noun.

Examples

Walking is a healthy exercise. [*Walking* is a gerund formed from the verb *walk,* and it is used as the *subject* of the sentence.]

The patient does appreciate my *caring.* [*Caring* is a gerund formed from the verb care. It is used as a *direct object* of the verb *does appreciate.*]

You can pass this course by *studying.* [The gerund *studying* is used as an *object of the preposition by.*]

The medical assistant's greatest reward is *learning.* [The gerund *learning* is used as a *predicate noun.* It follows the being verb *is.*]

A *gerund phrase* is a group of words consisting of a gerund and any other modifiers it may have. The gerund phrase, like a single gerund, functions as a noun.

Examples

Walking a mile is healthy exercise. [*Walking a mile* is a gerund phrase used as the *subject* of the sentence.]

The patient does appreciate *my caring.* [*My caring* is a gerund phrase used as a *direct object* of the verb *does appreciate.*]

You can pass this course by *studying daily.* [The gerund phrase *studying daily* is used as the *object of the preposition by.*]

The nurse's reward is *learning compassion.* [The gerund phrase *learning compassion* is used as a *predicate noun* following the being verb *is.*]

Note that both participles and gerunds end in *ing.* The difference is that a participle functions as an *adjective* and a *gerund* functions as a noun.

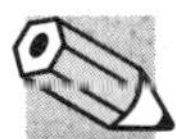

Practice 7-4

Identify the gerund phrase:

1. Selecting the correct antibiotic is crucial to this infection.
2. Calculating blood gases is an easy process.
3. Ears are examined using the otoscope.
4. Immunizing children can prevent certain diseases.
5. Checking equipment for accuracy is a skill acquired by experience.

6. Analyzing medical information helps to form a diagnosis.
7. Sterilizing instruments under pressurized steam is the most common method of sterilization.
8. The medical assistant was filing medical information.
9. Monitoring blood pressure can also be done in a home environment.
10. Weighing infants occurs shortly after they are born.

Infinitive Phrase

An infinitive is a verbal consisting of the present form of a verb usually preceded by the word *to.* It is generally used as a noun, and sometimes as an adjective or adverb.

Examples

Used as a subject	*To operate* would ease the pain.
Used as a direct object	The doctor wants *to operate.*
Used as a predicate noun	The decision was *to operate.*
Used as an adjective	The decision *to operate* was made by the patient.

Because both constructions include the word *to,* a clarification may be helpful in distinguishing between an infinitive and a prepositional phrase. An infinitive is a *verb* plus the word *to.* A prepositional phrase begins with the word *to* but is followed by a noun or pronoun as the object of the preposition.

Examples

Infinitive	*To smoke* causes lung damage.
Prepositional Phrase	Smoking causes damage *to the lungs.*

An *infinitive phrase* includes the infinitive and any subjects, objects, or modifiers. Like the infinitive itself, it generally functions as a noun, and sometimes as adjective or adverb.

Examples

Used as a noun	*To cure disease* became the goal of the scientist. [*To cure disease* is an infinitive phrase that functions as a subject.]
Used as a predicate noun	His plan is *to operate.* [*To operate* modifies plan. It comes after the being verb *is.*]
Used as an adjective	Medical researchers found a way *to solve the problem.* [*To solve the problem* describes the noun *way.*]
Used as an adverb	The medical assistant was encouraged *to help nurses.* [*To help nurses* modifies *was encouraged.*]

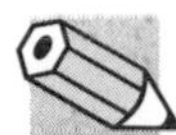

Practice 7-5

Identify the infinitive phrase in each sentence:

1. To attend the meeting was a real waste of time.
2. The nurse practitioner needs to analyze the test results.
3. A low fat diet given in small amounts helps to prevent cholecystitis.
4. Leukocytes help to protect the body from infection and tissue damage.
5. The medical assistant called the patients to confirm their appointments.
6. To excise the vermiform appendix is called an appendectomy.
7. X-rays are taken to validate any fractures.
8. The attending physician wanted to add I&O to the order.
9. The physician wanted to transfer the patient to the hospital.
10. The nutritionist's plan was to create healthy meals.

Appositive Phrase

An appositive phrase contains an appositive noun along with any modifying words. The phrase is placed next to the noun or pronoun it describes or renames. Commas are used to separate an appositive phrase.

Mike, *the class president,* called the meeting to order. [*The class president* renames Mike; *president* is the appositive noun modified by *the* and *class.*]

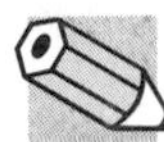

Practice 7-6

Identify the appositive phrase in each sentence:

1. A physician teaches microbiology, an important course for medical students.
2. Morphine, a drug used to control pain, is often given to cancer patients.
3. Nouns, a particular part of speech, name a person, place, thing, or idea.
4. Infection, an invasion of a pathogen, is the cause of many diseases.
5. Some protein foods, milk and fish, help repair tissues damaged by disease.
6. The Patient's Bill of Rights, a code of ethical standards, ensures that quality care be given to patients.

7. Xylocaine, a local anesthetic, was used to numb the wound.

8. The report contains a summary of the patient's ADL, activities of daily living.

9. The vital signs, temperature, pulse, respiration, and blood pressure, must be taken every hour.

10. The patient, Mrs. B in room 13, is on a special bland diet.

Clauses

A clause is a group of words that contains a subject and a verb within the structure of a sentence. Clauses are either independent or dependent.

Independent Clauses

An independent clause (also called a main clause) contains a subject and a verb and expresses a complete thought. An independent clause can stand by itself as a sentence.

Examples

The team wrote the patient's care plan.

The lecturer is an HMO representative.

Dependent Clauses

A dependent clause (also called a subordinate clause) contains a subject and verb, but does not express a complete thought and cannot stand alone as a sentence. A dependent clause has a sense of incompleteness about it. It sounds like something more should be said or written:

Examples

If you order your prescription today . . . [What about it? What happens if you order today? More information is needed to make this dependent clause complete the thought.]

that she didn't know [Know what?]

while she was in the hospital [What about it?]

To make a complete sentence, a dependent clause must be combined with an independent clause.

Examples

If you order your prescription today, you will get a discount.

There were many people at the medical conference *that she didn't know.*

The patient was too sick to read *while she was in the hospital.*

Dependent clauses are usually introduced by subordinating conjunctions or relative pronouns. Examples of subordinating conjunctions are *after, although, as, as if, as long as, as though, because, before, even though, how, if, in order that, provided that, rather than, since, so, so that, though, unless, until, when, whenever, where, wherever, whereas, whether,* and *while.* The relative pronouns are *which, that, who, whom,* or *whose.*

Examples

If a third party agrees to pay the medical bill, it must be in writing.

While the secretary was transcribing the report, the medical assistant answered incoming calls.

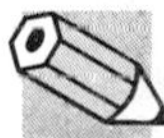

Practice 7-7

Identify the dependent clause in these sentences:

1. After the report is transcribed, erase the cassette.
2. When your doctor is sick, to whom do you go?
3. The medical assistant entered the data into the computer after the doctor visited the patient.
4. The information was entered into the computer when the nurse finished the procedures.
5. Medical assistants must use judgment when scheduling appointments that require more evaluation time.
6. The CPT code is assigned for services rendered after a patient has a procedure.
7. Demands for health care are increasing because people are living longer.
8. While the patient was in the hospital she developed Pseudomonas.
9. Autoimmune diseases are the cause of many chronic illnesses, when a person's self-antigens are damaged.
10. Sjögren's syndrome, because it is characterized by the dryness of the eyes and mouth, is an autoimmune disorder.

Different conjunctions introduce different types of dependent clauses, of which there are three: the *noun clause, adjective clause,* and *adverb clause.*

Noun Clause

The noun clause is a dependent clause that functions as a noun. It may be used as a subject, predicate noun, or direct object. Noun clauses are easy to detect because they are introduced by such words as *how, when, where, which, who (whoever), whom (whomever), whose, that, why, what,* or *whether.*

Examples

The problem is *that I am too dedicated to my profession.* [predicate noun after the verb *is*]

What the manager planned was a new hospital wing. [predicate noun after the verb *was*]

Do you know *what the emergency is?* [direct object]

The doctor didn't know *what to say.* [direct object]

Whoever locked the office door must open it. [subject]

What the manager planned was a new hospital wing. [subject]

Adjective Clause

An adjective clause is a dependent clause that tells about or describes a noun or pronoun. It is usually joined to a main clause by a relative pronoun: *which, that, who, whose,* or *whom.*

Examples

The interns saw the operation *Dr. Hartman performed.* [The adjective clause, *Dr. Hartman performed,* modifies the noun *operation.*]

The patient *whom the physician diagnosed with cancer* left suddenly. [The adjective clause, *whom the physician diagnosed with cancer,* modifies the noun *patient.*]

A medical assistant *whose name I can't remember* did a great job. [The adjective clause, *whose name I can't remember,* describes the noun *assistant.*]

Adverb Clause

An adverb clause functions as an adverb. It tells more about a verb, adjective, or another adverb. Adverb clauses are introduced by subordinating conjunctions such as *also, beside, for example, however, in addition to, instead, meanwhile, then,* and *therefore.* They answer the questions *how, when, why, where, how often, to what extent,* and *under what condition* about the verb.

Examples

List currency and coins *when you complete a deposit slip.* [The adverb clause, *when you complete a deposit slip,* modifies the verb *list.*]

Surgeons operate on weekends *if there is an emergency.* [The adverb clause, *if there is an emergency,* modifies the verb *operate.*]

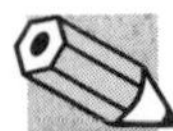

Practice 7-8

Identify the dependent clauses in each sentence:

1. Aspirin should not be used as an antipyretic with children because it may cause viral problems.
2. Phenylketonuria is a disease in which a hereditary enzyme is absent.
3. The staff was told when the patient arrived.
4. The electrocardiogram provides diagnostic information that the cardiologist needs.
5. When you finish, dispose of the syringes into the proper container.

Medical Spelling

Become familiar with the spelling of the following words:

appendectomy
artifacts
ascites
asymptomatic
audiogram
autoclave
autoimmunity
bronchiectasis
compatible
confidentiality
cystoscopy
demographics
diabetes insipidus
diabetes mellitus
dilemma
glomerulonephritis
glomerulus, glomeruli
glycosuria
guaiac
hematemesis
laryngitis
leukocytes
lithotripsy
mucous membrane
mucus
nephrectomy
oncology
palatine
Papanicolaou test
parenchyma
pathology
polyuria
prescription
Pseudomonas
Sjögren's syndrome
symptomatic
tinnitus
urology
varicella
vermiform appendix

Phrases Study Summary

Phrase: A group of words without a subject or predicate, which functions as a noun, adjective, or adverb in a sentence.

	Composition	Function	Example
Prepositional phrase	Begins with a preposition, plus nouns or pronouns and any modifiers.	Group of words that acts like a single modifier.	. . . valve *in the heart* . . . . . . parking lot *behind the hospital* . . . . . . time *at your earliest convenience*. . . .
Used as an adjective	Begins with a preposition, plus nouns or pronouns and modifiers.	Modifies a noun or pronoun. Answers *which one? what kind? how many?*	. . . the blood *in the heart* . . . . . . medicines *to cure infections* . . .
Used as an adverb	Begins with a preposition plus nouns or pronouns and any modifiers.	Modifies a verb, adjective, or other adverb. Answers *how? what? where? when? why? to what extent?*	The blood flowed *through the* aorta. The doctor operated *on weekends.* Nurses worked *around the clock.*

Verbal Phrases: A group of words including a verbal and its subject, object, complement, or modifiers that function as a noun, adjective, or adverb.

	Composition	Function	Example
Participial	Begins with verb ending in *ing* (present participle) or in *t, d, ed, en* (past participle).	Adjective	Nurses *dedicated to patient care* are unsung heroes. The report *containing the patient's history* was sent to another hospital.
Gerund	Begins with an *ing* verb and includes any modifiers.	Noun	*Eating healthy food* is an excellent habit. An excellent habit is *eating healthy food.*
Infinitive	Begins with *to,* plus present form of a verb and any modifiers.	Noun, predicate noun, or adverb	*To question* is a sign of intelligence. Numbers were put *into the computer.*

Appositive Phrase: An appositive noun and any modifiers that describes or renames a noun: "The Ethics Committee, *ten members strong,* met yesterday." "Terminology, *a study of words,* is essential in health professions."

Clauses Study Summary

Clause: A group of words containing a subject and verb. Independent clauses contain a subject and a verb, express a complete thought, and can exist alone as a sentence. Dependent clauses contain a subject and a verb, but do not express a complete thought and cannot exist alone in a sentence.

Dependent clauses are introduced by subordinating conjunctions and relative pronouns:

Subordinating Conjunctions	***Relative Pronouns***
after, although, as, as if, as long as, as though, because, before, even though, how, if, in order that, provided that, rather than, since, so, so that, that, though, unless, until, when, whenever, where, wherever, whereas, whether, while	*which, that, who, whom, whose*

Function	**Identifier**	**Example**
Noun used as a subject, predicate noun, or direct object	Introduced by *how, when, where, which, who, whoever, whom, whomever, whose, that, why, what, whether.*	The wheelchair is *what I ordered.* I know *how you are feeling.*
Adjective used to tell *which one* or *what kind.*	Often introduced by a relative pronoun: *which, that, who, whose, whom.*	That was the house *where Dr. Brown lived.* Supplies, *which were ordered in May,* have not arrived yet.
Adverb used to tell about a verb, adjective, or another adverb.	Introduced by *also, because, beside, for example, however, if, in addition to, instead, meanwhile, then, therefore.*	She practices *because she wants to be a better pianist.* *If you discover a fire,* ring the alarm immediately.

Skills Review

Identify the italicized words as a phrase or a clause:

1. Studying is essential *while attending college courses.* ____________________
2. A pregnant woman can give diseases *to her unborn child.* ____________________
3. Medical information is kept confidential *unless a release form is signed.* ____________________
4. Weight varies *according to one's exercise patterns.* ____________________
5. *After she completed the form,* she proofread it for errors. ____________________
6. The journal printed last month had an article *about cancer research.* ____________________
7. *Although vital signs were stable,* the patient remained *in surgical recovery.* ____________________

8. The doctor increased the dosage *because the patient would be more comfortable.* ___________________

9. A physician, *with years of experience,* performed the operation. ___________________

10. Six members *of the ethics committee* went to the seminar. ___________________

11. *When you know the test results,* give me a call. ___________________

12. The man consulted a specialist *for neck and head pain.* ___________________

13. After he was *covered with an additional blanket,* the patient felt warmer. ___________________

14. We have time *to bandage the wound.* ___________________

15. Chris's goal is to do research *in the medical profession.* ___________________

Underline any phrases within the paragraph:

Education is a vital service to both patients and physicians. Patients often experience anxiety over health concerns. Health-care providers must work to foster patient confidence and trust. The medical assistant tries to establish a rapport between the patient and physician. Medical assistants often suggest to patients that they prepare questions for the doctor. The assistant may also alert the physician of a patient's health concerns. Information about fees, office hours, insurance, office policies, and Medicare should also be readily available. In this manner, the medical assistant performs a vital service to both patients and physicians. The services of medical assistants are a great value to the medical profession.

Underline any clauses within these paragraphs:

Health-care providers must educate patients who need specific health information. Patient education is an important function of the allied health professional. When a professional deals with patients, state medical information in clear, concise language that patients can understand. Gathering additional information such as pictures, pamphlets, films, and community resources is also helpful.

Follow an outline when planning patient education. An outline should include interesting topics. Share the teaching plan with a physician who may add additional information. After completing patient education, evaluate the session's effectiveness. Health-care providers who educate patients about health issues provide valuable information that could help the patient throughout life.

Rewrite these sentences and place the phrase or clause next to the word it modifies:

1. That I wrote the doctor's report was lost. ____________________
2. When the operation would begin Christine asked. ____________________
3. Where patients can hear them nurses should not talk. ____________________
4. The record is called minutes of the meeting. ____________________
5. Attention to details will speed delivery when ordering. ____________________
6. What the prognosis was, Mark didn't hear. ____________________
7. Out the window I looked for the incoming ambulance. ____________________
8. In a cast Val had her arm. ____________________
9. Who had a heart attack the doctor visited the patient. ____________________
10. People live longer who exercise. ____________________

Circle the correctly spelled word in each line:

1.	delemma	dilemma	dilema	dilimma
2.	compitible	compatable	compatibel	compatible
3.	appendectomy	apendectomy	appendactomy	appindectomy
4.	confidintiality	confidentiality	confedentiality	confidenteality
5.	mucos	mukus	mucus	mucuus
6.	patology	pothology	pathology	patholgy
7.	simptomatic	symtomatic	sympamatic	symptomatic
8.	prescriptions	priscriptions	prescreptions	perscriptions
9.	tinitus	tinnitus	tinnetus	tinnitis
10.	laringitis	larygetis	laryngites	laryngitis

Translate medical abbreviations using a medical dictionary or appendix.

1. q. ____________________
2. q.i.d. ____________________
3. PVC ____________________
4. q.3 h. ____________________
5. q.n.s. ____________________
6. RBC ____________________
7. R/O ____________________
8. Rx ____________________
9. RLQ ____________________
10. rehab ____________________

Chapter 8

Sentences

Objectives

Upon completion of this chapter, the student should be able to:

- identify the three basic types of sentence structures
- recognize the four classifications of sentences according to their purpose
- identify the factors that cause ineffective sentences
- utilize the factors that contribute to the effectiveness of sentences
- spell various medical terms
- translate various medical abbreviations

This chapter explains how to arrange parts of speech, phrases, and clauses into clear, effective sentences.

The writing style used in the medical profession is unique. When medical personnel document data, it is usually written without regard to sentence structure. Information is jotted down in abbreviations, words, and symbols. However, when this information is translated into formal letters or reports, correct sentence structure is absolutely necessary.

Examples

Medical documentation: Pt. is scheduled for TURP

Sentence translation: The patient is scheduled for transurethral resection of the prostate.

Medical documentation: Dx is CHF

Sentence translation: The diagnosis is congestive heart failure.

Components of Sentences

A sentence expresses a complete thought. To be grammatically correct and express a complete thought, every sentence must have two basic parts: a subject and a predicate. The subject is the part about which or whom something is said. The predicate is the part that tells about the subject. The simple subject is the main noun or pronoun in the sentence; the simple predicate is referred to as the *verb.*

Simple Subject	***Simple Predicate (Verb)***
Medication	cures.
Physicians	examine.
Payment	received.

To find the subject of the sentence, locate the verb and ask the question *who?* or *what?* about it.

Verb is *cures. What* cures? Medication cures. *Medication* is the *subject.*

Verb is *examine. Who* examines? Physicians examine. Physic*ians* is the *subject.*

Verb is *received. What* was received? Payment received. *Payment* is the *subject.*

Subjects and predicates may be compound. A compound subject consists of two or more subjects connected by the conjunction *and* or *or*. A compound subject has the same verb. A compound predicate has two or more verbs linked by the conjunction *and, or,* or *but.* The compound predicate has the same subject.

Compound Subject	**Compound Predicate**
Medication and rest cure.	Medications *cure or arrest diseases.*
Physicians and nurses document.	Physicians *document and dictate.*
Payment and claims received.	Payment *received and stamped.*

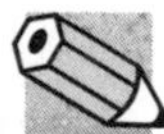

Practice 8-1

Identify the subject of each sentence by asking who? or what? about the verb (predicate):

1. The operation was cancelled. ____________________
2. The major ethical and legal concern related to the medical record is confidentiality. ____________________
3. The patient owns the information in the medical record. ____________________
4. The physician owns the medical record itself. ____________________
5. The patient's written consent and physician's approval are needed to release medical information. ____________________
6. Signed authorization is not required for a subpoena. ____________________
7. The server of the subpoena gives the office a check to cover the processing costs. ____________________
8. If information wasn't recorded, it wasn't done. ____________________
9. Entries in a medical record are unalterable. ____________________
10. A breach of confidentiality has legal implications. ____________________

Sentence Structure

The three sentence structures are simple, compound, and complex.

Simple Sentence

A simple sentence has one independent clause.

Examples

Sutures are surgical stitches.

Patient records are known as charts.

Compound Sentence

A compound sentence contains two or more independent clauses.

Examples

Medical asepsis involves procedures to reduce microorganisms and handwashing is the first step in the process.

The appointment schedule was booked solid; therefore, only emergencies were accepted.

Complex Sentence

A complex sentence has one independent clause and one or more dependent clauses.

Examples

When preparing for surgical asepsis, the objective is to eliminate all microorganisms.

Bookkeeping and banking are two important responsibilities when a medical assistant works in an office setting.

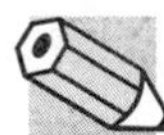

Practice 8-2

Identify the sentences as either simple, compound, or complex.

1. Many supplies in the doctor's office are disposable and many are made of surgical steel for autoclaving. ____________________

2. When one is preparing for surgical asepsis, the objective is to eliminate all microorganisms. ____________________

3. Autoclaving is the most common method of sterilizing. ____________________

4. Keep charts neat. ____________________

5. When filing space is limited, computer storage may be necessary. ____________________

6. Sterile solutions are often required during surgical procedures. ____________________

Classifications of Sentences

Sentences are classified in four ways according to what they do: declarative, imperative, exclamatory, and interrogative.

Declarative Sentences

Most sentences are declarative because they make known (*declare)* some type of information or statement. Declarative sentences end with a period (.).

Examples

The medical assistant is responsible for filing.

The diagnosis is influenza.

A differential diagnosis is given when there are other possible diagnoses.

Pulse oximetry revealed an oxygen saturation of 83%.

The record will be organized according to the needs of the physicians.

Imperative Sentences

Imperative sentences give a command or make a request. In an imperative sentence, the word *you* is understood as the subject, even though it is not written. Imperative sentences end with a period (.).

Examples

Transcribe the History and Physical in full block form.

Make the margins one inch on either side of the report.

Photocopy the correspondence and file it.

Fax this consultation letter to Dr. Villes.

Make the follow-up appointment in one week.

Interrogative Sentences

Interrogative sentences ask direct questions and end with a question mark (?).

Examples

Did you include the name of the patient and the reason for the appointment?

What is the etiology of that disease?

Do you know the difference between exocrine and endocrine?

What is OSHA?

How are charting errors changed or corrected?

Exclamatory Sentences

Exclamatory sentences express strong emotions and end with an exclamation point (!).

Examples

The patient is in cardiac arrest!

STAT!

Call 911!

Prepare the operating room now!

Look at the size of that tumor!

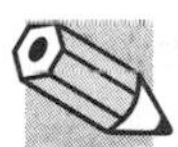

Practice 8-3

State whether the following sentences are declarative, imperative, exclamatory, or interrogative:

1. Does your family have a history of cancer? ____________________
2. Medical forms will be processed if signed by both parties. ____________________
3. Write your signature on this form, please. ____________________
4. Epinephrine STAT! ____________________
5. The patient has been examined for hospital admission. ____________________
6. Leave a message at the tone. ____________________
7. Have you scheduled the operating room yet? ____________________
8. Eliminate the allergens to reduce the asthma attacks. ____________________
9. Anxiety is a normal response to surgery. ____________________
10. Get the oxygen! ____________________

> *There's almost no more beautiful sight than a simple declarative sentence.*
>
> William Zinsser

Ineffective Sentences

In addition to having good writing skills, it is essential for the health professional to be able to detect poorly constructed sentences. A poorly constructed sentence is one that disrupts the smooth flow of a clear message. Two common constructions that cause ineffective sentences are fragmented sentences and run-on sentences.

The Fragmented Sentence

Sentences that do not express a complete thought are called *fragmented sentences* because some necessary information is omitted. Fragmented sentences occur when a phrase or a dependent clause is erroneously punctuated as though it were a complete sentence.

Examples

Because of medical staff absenteeism.

If you want to stay healthy.

Medical x-rays indicate.

Medications in the locked closet.

The preceding examples are dependent clauses. Additional information must be added to make complete sentences. Notice that fragmented sentences may contain a subject and verb; however, they depend on other clauses to give meaning to the sentence.

Examples

Because of medical staff absenteeism, everything was behind schedule.

If you want to stay healthy, drink more water and exercise daily.

Medical x-rays indicate an abnormality in the neck.

Medications in the locked closet need to be distributed.

> *Edit, revise, and proofread each sentence until it is clear and complete.*

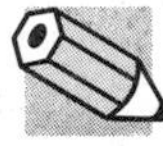

Practice 8-4

State whether these sentences are complete or fragmented:

1. One of the physicians at the hospital. ____________________
2. Recording each patient's medication. ____________________
3. Common charting terminology. ____________________
4. If you see a light. ____________________
5. Give 50 mg of morphine SC stat. ____________________
6. The lab technician doesn't seem to care. ____________________
7. Use plastic gloves for aseptic reasons. ____________________
8. Decontaminate work surfaces. ____________________

9. Whenever the time came for him to operate. ____________________

10. Used for the urine culture. ____________________

Run-on Sentences

A more common sentence error than the fragmented sentence is the run-on sentence, where two or more sentences run together as one. A run-on sentence occurs in three ways:

1. A comma is used between two sentences instead of a period. This misuse is called a comma splice.

   The patient can waive confidentiality, confidentiality can be overruled through a court order or subpoena.

2. A semicolon (;) is used between two sentences instead of a period.

   The patient can waive confidentiality; confidentiality can be overruled through a court order or a subpoena.

3. A coordinating conjunction (and, but, or) is omitted from between two complete sentences.

   The patient can waive confidentiality—confidentiality can be overruled by a court order or subpoena.

> *A run-on sentence has too many ideas and not enough punctuation.*

Practice 8-5

Identify the following sentences as complete or run-on:

1. Have you read the chapter on confidentiality insuring protected communication between the patient and the provider regarded as privileged information?

   ____

2. Where can the doctor be he was here a minute ago? ____________________

3. Let's go over medical terms before taking the test. ____________________

4. An unintentional tort is when there is an omission or a committed act that a reasonably prudent person would or would not do in a given situation. ____________________

5. A frozen section is a technique used to prepare a biopsy sample for examination.

   ____

6. Nonfeasance, malfeasance, malpractice, and criminal negligence are professionally wrong and are types of negligence. ____________________

7. The autopsy results are in there will be a special report. ____________________

8. Evidence that points to "let the thing speak for itself" strongly implies negligence is called "res ipsa loquitur." ____________________

9. Communicable diseases are usually reported to the community and district health departments. ____________________

10. The Joint Commission of the Accreditation of Healthcare Organization (JCAHO) accredits health-care institutions. ____________________

Poor punctuation is the main cause of run-on sentences. Run-on sentences may be corrected in four ways:

1. Separate the two complete compound sentences with a period.

   The M.A. uses a computer to schedule appoints. It also stores information.

2. Separate the complete thoughts by using a coordinating conjunction (*and, but,* or *or).*

   The M.A. uses a computer to schedule appointments, and it also stores information.

3. Separate the two complete thoughts with a semicolon.

   The M.A. uses a computer to schedule appointments; it also stores information.

4. Make one of the independent clauses into a phrase or dependent clause.

   The M.A. uses a computer to schedule appointments *that also stores information.*

By not using a period, semicolon, or conjunction, one sentence is permitted to run into another. Carelessness rather than a lack of understanding more likely causes this type of error.

Examples

Run-on	I took her vital signs I marked the results on the patient's chart. [No punctuation mark or coordinating conjunction used between the two complete sentences.]
Correct	I took her vital signs. I marked the results on the patient's chart. [A period separates the two sentences.]
Correct	After I took her vital signs, I marked the results on the patient's chart. [Revised to make a single sentence with a dependent and independent clause.]
Run-on	I took her vital signs, I marked the results on the patient's chart. [A comma is used in place of a period.]
Correct	I took her vital signs, and I marked the results on the patient's chart. [Added a coordinating conjunction.]

Effective Sentences

Writing for medical professionals is very different from other professions. A person's reason for writing greatly influences the tone or manner in which words are expressed. A novelist uses multiple words to create settings, establish moods, and express emotions. An historian concentrates on exact times, cultures, and the cause and effect of events. A poet uses metaphors, rhythm, and rhyme. Medical writers use abbreviations, codes, and phrases unique to their situations. Note the difference in style between a novelist and a medical professional:

Novelist

How glad she was to see her children! She wept for pleasure when she felt their little arms clasping her; their hard, ruddy cheeks pressing against her own glowing cheeks. She looked into their faces with hungry eyes that could not be satisfied with looking.

[Kate Chopin, *The Awakening*]

Medical Professional

Patient experiences no motion in the back. Range of motion of the hips is within normal limits and painless. There is only a +1 dorsalis pedis on the right; otherwise, there are no peripheral pulses present. There is marked coldness of both feet.

[Diehl and Fordney, *Medical Typing and Transcribing*]

Many elements contribute to the effectiveness of good sentence structure. Four of these elements are covered in this chapter: parallel structure, conciseness, word choices, and positive statements.

Parallel Structure

Parallel sentence structure requires that words, phrases, and clauses be expressed in the same grammatical structure. A sentence reads more smoothly when the writer takes time to express parallel ideas in the same form. Parallel structure happens when one part of speech, phrase, or clause, matches another word (or words) that is used in the same manner, for example,

a noun with a noun	*doctors* and *nurses*
an adjective with an adjective	*red* and *green* lights
an infinitive with an infinitive	*to* speak and *to* listen
a gerund with a gerund	*climbing* and *reaching*

Examples

Nonparallel	Dr. Spencer is *trustworthy* and a *gynecologist.* [*Trustworthy* is an adjective and *gynecologist* is a noun.]
Parallel	Dr. Spencer is a *surgeon* and a *gynecologist.* Two nouns.
Parallel	Dr. Spencer is trustworthy and honest. [two adjectives]
Nonparallel	The medical assistant's tasks are *transcribing* and *to file.* [*Transcribing* is a gerund and *to file* is an infinitive.]
Parallel	A medical assistant's tasks are *transcribing* and *filing.* [two gerunds]
Parallel	A medical assistant's tasks are *to transcribe* and *to file.* [two infinitives]
Nonparallel	The nurse is *knowledgeable, sincere,* and *she is dedicated.*
Parallel	The nurse is *knowledgeable, sincere,* and *dedicated.*

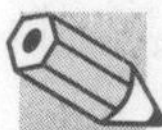

Practice 8-6

Identify these sentences as parallel or nonparallel:

1. The supervisor's responsibilities include supervising programs, writing grants, and to schedule work hours for the medical assistants. ____________________

2. Use abbreviations when charting and entering the information into the computer. ____________________

3. The patient underwent an MRI, an X-ray, and blood test. ____________________

4. The patient education was interesting and of knowledge. ____________________

5. The doctor proofread the History and Physical quickly and thoroughly. ____________________

6. I want an appointment for next week, rather than putting it off until next month. ____________________

7. Go to the elevator, get off on the third floor, turn left, and you will enter room 306. ____________________

8. Ann purchased a computer, a color printer, and she also bought a modem. ____________________

9. To update the office, the medical secretary wanted to get new equipment and refurbish old wooden desks. ____________________

10. She is a well-trained, sensitive physician and you can rely on her opinion. ____________________

Conciseness

Conciseness is the hallmark of medical documentation. Conciseness is expressing a lot of information in a few words. More words are not necessarily better. Sentences should not be cluttered with unnecessary words.

Examples

Wordy	The black and blue mark is on the right lower leg.
Concise	The hematoma is on the right lower leg.
Wordy	If you think you want more information, don't hesitate to call.
Concise	Call me for more information.
Wordy	The purpose of this letter is to acknowledge the receipt of your medical payment.
Concise	Thank you for your remittance.

Wordy	We received your check for the full amount.
Concise	We received the balance in full.
Wordy	The patient has difficulty breathing.
Concise	The patient has dyspnea.
Wordy	To the best of my knowledge, we did all we could do for the patient.
Concise	We did all we could for the patient.

> *A sentence should contain no unnecessary words, a paragraph no unnecessary sentences, for the same reason that a drawing should have no unnecessary line and a machine no unnecessary part.*
>
> William Strunk, Jr.

Wordy expressions can be replaced by concise words:

as a result	therefore
at this time, at this point in time	now, currently
bring to a conclusion	conclude, end
cognizant of the fact	know
due to the fact that	because
during the month of	during
each and every	each
enclosed please find	I am enclosing
lend credence to the report	lend support
many eccentricities	many behaviors
peruse the document	read the document
I would appreciate it if	please
in regard to	regarding, concerning
in some cases	sometimes
in reference to the subject matter	regarding
in the near future	soon
it has come to our attention	we learned
it is incumbent on	it is your duty
of primary importance	significant
please be advised that	know
regarding the matter of	regarding

Practice 8-7

Make these sentences more concise:

1. The patient is not expected until some time in late July. ____________________

2. You are eligible for Medicare because of the fact of your age. ____________________

3. I shall be extremely glad to be of assistance to you. ____________________

4. The pharmacy makes deliveries of customer's medications for a charge that amounts to $7.00 per delivery. ____________________

5. The group moves to negotiate acceptance of the physician's plan.
____

6. During the month of April, my health premiums increased by the amount of 5%.
____

7. All medical assistants were asked to familiarize themselves with the new procedures.
____

8. It is estimated by security that the office was broken into about 8:30 p.m.
____

9. When a nurse finds it necessary to rest her weary bones, she packs up and goes on what is called a vacation. ____________________

10. Enclosed please find a check in the amount of $100. ____________________

To be concise also means to reduce the length of sentences. Writing shorter sentences means using fewer words. Ten or fifteen words per sentence is about average. Be careful of sentences that run longer than two typed lines. Shorten lengthy sentences by adding periods and making two or more sentences out of one. For example,

Lengthy Sentence	The gallbladder was edematous and somewhat thick-walled, with a stone lodged in the cystic duct of the gallbladder, measuring about 1.0 cm in diameter, but there were no filling defects and there was good emptying of the contrast medium into the duodenum.
Revision	The gallbladder was edematous and somewhat thick-walled. It contained a 1.0 cm stone lodged in the cystic duct of the gallbladder, which had no filling defects. There was good emptying of the contrast medium into the duodenum.

Eliminate unnecessary words. Write to express, not impress.

On the other hand, too many short sentences could be boring:

Short Sentences	Heather Adams is an 83-year-old woman. She also looks young for her age. She has a history of heart problems. She refused medication. It makes her dizzy. There are also occasional accidents from incontinence. Also diarrhea. X-rays were ordered.
Varied Sentences	Heather Adams is an 83-year-old woman with a history of heart problems. She refuses medication because it makes her dizzy. The patient experiences incontinence and diarrhea. X-rays were ordered.

Another way to be concise is to change a dependent clause into either a phrase, an appositive, or a single word.

Phrase (a group of words without a subject or predicate)

Working medical staff [gerund phrase]

After the operation [prepositional phrase]

To get an early start [infinitive phrase]

Troubled by headaches [participial phrase]

Appositive (a word or group of words that renames)

John, who is the physical therapist = John, the physical therapist

Single Word

That had been canceled = canceled

Examples

Clause	The biopsy *that came to the pathology laboratory* was not scheduled for today.
Phrase	The biopsy *from the pathology lab* was not scheduled for today.
Clause	*After you graduate*, you are eligible for the certification exam.
Phrase	*After graduation*, you are eligible for the certification exam.
Clause	Her two nurses, *one of whom is Joan and the other Bill,* took care of her.
Appositive	Her two nurses, *Joan and Bill,* took care of her.
Phrase	Angry, upset patients need to be handled *in a positive manner.*
Single Word	Angry, upset patients need to be handled *positively.*
Clause	Allow the patient *who is angry* to express his feelings
Single Word	Allow the *angry* patient to express his feelings.

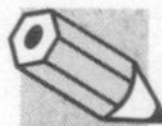

Practice 8-8

Keep the meaning of these sentences, but make them more concise:

1. In chart notes, some doctors write in longhand that is hard to read.
   ____

2. The patient had herpes zoster at a young age and recovered nicely.
   ____

3. The patient is alert, holding the right section of his arm at times during the exam.
   ____

4. Prompt diagnosis and treatment comes from early recognition of signs and symptoms.
   ____

5. When original materials are used in a report, credit must be given to the author in a footnote. ____________________

Diction

Diction refers to the writer's choice of words and how those words are used in writing. Diction makes the difference between a clear style and a weak, vague style. The intended audience usually determines the type of diction. Among the types that have no place in medical documentation are colloquial, vague, slang, and unfamiliar words.

Some writers feel that using long or unfamiliar words make a good impression. Although these words have their merit, medical documentation is not the place to impress.

Examples

The patient's *idiosyncrasies* irritated her condition.

The patient's *behavior* irritated her condition.

Peruse the medical report before you make any comment.

Read the medical report before you make any comment.

Slang is a new or old expression that contains colorful words and expressions that take on new meaning. Phrases like, *don't bug me, it's cool, in the swim, off the wall, it's not my bag* are examples of slang. Colloquialisms are informal words and phrases used in everyday conversation: *globs, lots and lots, all revved up, boondocks, keel over,* and *been there–done that.*

Examples

The patient is *off the wall.*

Medical research *is not my thing*

The new medical equipment is real *groovy.*

Another trap to avoid in writing effective sentences is the use of vague words or phrases. Vagueness is expressing oneself unclearly. Like slang and colloquialisms, vague words have no place in medical documentation. Recording that a patient received medication without the name or dosage of the drug opens the door to all kinds of problems. Can you imagine the consequences if a medical assistant failed to document that a patient's *right* hand was the source of pain? Be specific with the facts. Assume nothing in medical reporting. Use specific words over vague words or wordy expressions.

Examples

Vague	The patient wasn't feeling well.
Specific	The patient complained of abdominal pain. His skin was cool, pale, and moist.
Vague	The medication was given before bedtime.
Specific	A.S.A. 500 mg was given H.S.
Vague	The head nurse supervised the project.
Specific	Ellen Barker, the head nurse, supervised the Ethics Project.
Vague	Call me some time during the day.
Specific	Call me between 1:00 and 2:00 p.m. on Wednesday.

> *The difference between the right word and the nearly right word is the same as that between lightning and the lightning bug.*
>
> Mark Twain

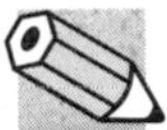

Practice 8-9

Underline the sentence in each pair that provides specific information:

1. A. What do you expect from someone who comes from the boondocks?

   B. Make the appointment on Wednesday at 3:15 p.m.

2. A. The physician informed the Board of Directors about the financial situation.

   B. Last night, the patient had lots and lots of pain and discomfort.

3. A. You and I think along the same lines.

   B. The moral issue about confidentiality was discussed at the meeting.

4. A. Credit was given to Dr. Sullivan for his consultation report.

   B. Although many suggestions were good, some were very far out.

5. A. The patient could care less about what medication to take.

   B. I appreciate the effort you put into fund raising.

Positive Statements

To write more effective sentences, use positive statements instead of negative ones. Write what can be done rather than what cannot be done. A positive tone creates an environment of efficiency, acceptance, and professionalism. Notice how these negative sentences were changed to positive sentences:

Negative	Your medication isn't due until 3 p.m.
Positive	Your medication is due at 3 p.m.
Negative	Why didn't you clean the wound before applying bacitracin?
Positive	Clean the wound well before applying the bacitracin.
Negative	The medication isn't in stock right now.
Positive	We expect to receive the medication tomorrow.
Negative	You did not sign the release form.
Positive	Please sign the release form.

Negative sentences, like those used in the previous examples, contain some form of the word *not* (*nor, never, no*). Some sentences may also convey a negative tone even without using *not*:

Negative	Doctors are like God.
Positive	Doctors are human like everyone else.
Negative	Get it right the first time.
Positive	I'll take my time and do it well.
Negative	What if I lose my job?
Positive	If I lose my job, I'll find a better one.

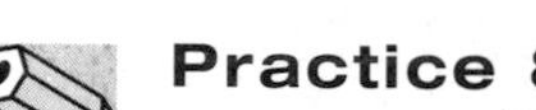

Practice 8-10

Change these negative sentences to positive ones:

1. Most people never change. ____________________
2. I feel miserable. ____________________
3. I can't be good at everything. ____________________
4. When things go wrong, I'm to blame. ____________________
5. My supervisor refused to give me a raise. ____________________
6. Do not refund the money. ____________________
7. The doctor's office isn't open after 5 p.m. ____________________
8. Do not finish the report until after your vacation. ____________________

9. You won't be satisfied with the quality of care in that hospital. ____________

10. Don't think twice about calling the doctor. ____________

Medical Spelling

Become familiar with the spelling of the following words:

absenteeism
allergens
alleviate
anaphylaxis
anticoagulant
apprehension
asepsis
astringent
authorization
communicable
correspondence
culture
dyspnea, dyspneic
electrode
endocrine
epinephrine
etiology
exocrine
hematocrit
hemoglobin
idiopathic
immunization
implications
influenza
isopropyl
lithotomy
mammogram
manipulation
negligence
oximetry
Papanicolaou test
pathogens
precautions
resuscitation
scissors
subpoena
technician
temperature
vacuum
waive

Sentence Study Summary

Sentence	Subject (Simple or Compound)	Complete Subject	Simple Predicate (Verb)	Complete Predicate
My sister, Ethel, is a technician	Ethel (simple subject)	My sister, Ethel	is	is a technician.
Free dental care was given to children.	care (simple subject)	free dental care	was	was given to the children.
The hurricane and wind destroyed many houses and trees.	hurricane and wind (compound subject)	The hurricane and wind	destroyed	destroyed many houses and trees.

Sentence Structure

Simple Sentence	Contains one independent clause.	The disease was contagious.
Compound Sentence	Contains two or more independent clauses.	The disease was contagious but precautions were taken.
Complex Sentence	Contains one independent clause and one dependent clause.	Careful handwashing reduces the spread of contagious disease when done properly.

Classifications of Sentences

Declarative	Makes a statement, used more than any other type, and ends in a period: "This doctor seldom asks for a copayment."
Imperative	Gives a command, makes a request, and ends in a period. The subject *you* is understood: "Give the patient medicine." "Don't forget your appointment."
Exclamatory	Expresses strong feelings, and ends with an exclamation point: "Get to the ER quickly!"
Interrogative	Asks a question and ends with a question mark: "What is my temperature?" "When are you flying to France?"

Ineffective Sentences

Fragmented	Does not express a complete thought and occurs when a phrase is considered as a sentence: "involuntary shaking," "under medical care," "who are known to have hemophilia."
Run-on	When a comma or semicolon is used between two sentences instead of a period, or a coordinating conjunction is omitted from between two sentences: "Chart notes are formal or informal; physicians take them when they see a patient." "The abdomen is flat without scars bowel sounds are normative." "Make an entry in the chart, do the entry correctly."

Characteristics of Effective Sentences

Parallel structure	Two or more sentence elements of equal rank expressed similarly: "Water skiing is as challenging as to dive." [not parallel] "Water skiing is as challenging as diving." (parallel]
Conciseness	Avoiding wordiness and sentences that are too long: "We were sitting in seats that were close to the stage." [wordy] "We were sitting close to the stage." [concise]
Appropriate diction	Clear expression through the choice of words and how they are used in a sentence: "The meeting is in the afternoon." [vague] "The team meeting is at 3:30 p.m." [precise]
Positive statements	Affirmative expression: "I can't perform that procedure." [negative] "I'll refer you to a physician who does that procedure." [positive]

Skills Review

Complete these fragmented sentences:

1. For medical coverage to continue. ______________
2. Your medical insurance representative. ______________
3. The results from your MRI. ______________
4. An adjustment made to the patient's claim. ______________
5. People with job-related illnesses. ______________
6. A variety of medical insurance plans in the United States. ______________
7. Medications covered by insurance. ______________
8. Diagnoses were recorded ______________
9. Her history was recorded ______________
10. An earlier appointment was made ______________

Select the best sentence from among the three choices:

1. A. I see an arrhythmia on the telemetry call the cardiologist

   B. I see an arrhythmia on the telemetry, call the cardiologist.

   C. I see an arrhythmia on the telemetry. Call the cardiologist.

2. A. The person is dyspneic, she needs oxygen.

   B. The person is dyspneic; she needs oxygen.

   C. The person is dyspneic she needs oxygen.

3. A. The biopsy is tomorrow I hope for good news.

   B. The biopsy is tomorrow, therefore, I hope for good news.

   C. The biopsy is tomorrow and I hope for good news.

4. A. The hospital wing is closed repairs are being made.

   B. The hospital wing is closed because repairs are being made.

   C. The hospital is closed, repairs are being made.

5. A. A nurse expresses compassion when she works with her patients.

   B. A nurse expresses compassion when he works with his patients.

   C. Nurses express compassion when they work with their patients.

6. A. Medicine is a service to mankind.

   B. Medicine is a service to womankind.

   C. Medicine is a service to humankind.

7. A. Doctors are available for consultation around the clock.

   B. Doctors are available for 24-hour consultation.

   C. Doctors are available night and day for consultation.

8. A. The lab technician is on the first floor.

   B. The lab technician on the first floor.

   C. The lab technician on the first floor right.

9. A. The side effects of the medicine are headaches and vomiting.

   B. The side effects of the medicine are headaches and an upset stomach.

   C. The side effects of the medicine are vomiting and upset stomach.

10. A. Implants could be placed in the next 3 to 4 months under those circumstances as described above here.

    B. Implants could be placed in the next three to four months as described above.

    C. Under these circumstances as described above here in the next 3 to 4 months implants could be placed.

Improve these sentences. (Many of them were obtained from actual doctor's reports.)

1. Dr. Archie placed these implants in her office. ____________________

2. The procedure was successful and the patient left the operating room in excellent condition. ____________________

3. If you should have any questions or comments please don't hesitate to call me.
   ____

4. The doctor needs a lawyer for his malpractice case. ____________________

5. Dr. Villes left Chicago with one hygienist that did not have a complete schedule. ____________________

6. To the best of my knowledge, the biopsy was negative. ____________________

7. To the best of my knowledge, you are now 40 years of age and are passing a magical mark in your life. ____________________

8. The patient moved slowly. She moved along the corridor, She used her walker. ____________________

9. I would like to thank you for your ongoing confidence and wish you a pleasant spring. ____________________

10. After the operation, bring the patient to the next room over in the recovery room. ____________________

11. He has raised questions as to the feasibility and appropriateness of doing this given the fact that he will be 90 years old in the next few months. ____________________

12. The above patient was in our office for preventative measures and appears to be generally stable. ____________________

13. The problem was here yesterday and it will be here tomorrow unless you do something about it today. ____________________

14. If my secretary has not called you yet, please call her and schedule a 45 minute consultation. ____________________

15. The concept was unique and different from any in existence. ____________________

16. This communication is to notify you that your results to your blood chemistry are normal. ____________________

17. An updated set of radiographs has been sent, which are enclosed for review and your permanent file. ____________________

18. Do not jargonize language in a medical report. ____________________

19. The patient was recently in our office and is generally doing well at that time. ____________________

20. He reported no change in the medical history and the examination was WNL. ____________________

21. Having completed the osteotomy a guide pin was placed and two additional osteotomies were completed using the drill. ____________________

22. The patient drinks several beers a day and occasionally a cigar or cigarette.

    ____

23. Hot compresses to the right hand. ____________________

24. Hygiene was carefully enforced. ____________________

25. Bone loss was generally 30% and it was thought to be generally 10%.

    ____

26. Pathogens flow through the air with the greatest of ease. ____________________

27. Having approximated the flaps and using sutures it was noted the patient was in good condition. ____________________

28. Xylocaine 2% without epinephrine was administered into the tissues because of the patients previous problem with increased heart rate with epinephrine.

    ____

29. The patient is to follow up with Dr. Valerie Christopher two days after discharge.

    ____

30. Patient was draped, in the usual manner, and brought to the operating room.

    ____

Circle the correctly spelled word in each line:

1. aprehension	apprihension	apprehension	apprehision
2. absenteism	abcenteism	absentiism	absenteeism
3. epiniphrine	epinefrin	epinephrine	epunephrin
4. dyspneic	dispnyic	dyspnic	dispneic
5. implications	implycations	immplications	immplecations
6. papnicoloau	Papanicolaou	Paipicolaou	papanicolaou
7. anaphilaxis	anaphilaxis	anafilaxis	anaphylaxis
8. communicable	comunicable	cummunicable	comunecable
9. rescitation	resuscitation	resussitation	ressusitation
10. oximetry	auximitry	oxemitry	auximitre

Translate medical abbreviations using a medical dictionary or appendix.

1. sed. rt. ____________________
2. SOB ____________________
3. stat ____________________
4. Sx ____________________
5. sp. gr. ____________________
6. t.i.d. ____________________
7. TURP ____________________
8. U/A ____________________
9. URI ____________________
10. UTI ____________________

Chapter 9

Punctuation

Objectives

Upon completion of this chapter, the student should be able to:

- apply the appropriate punctuation marks to the ends of sentences
- recognize when to use periods other than at the ends of sentences
- use internal sentence punctuation correctly
- understand when to use parentheses, dashes, hyphens, apostrophes, italics, and quotation marks
- spell various medical terms
- translate various medical abbreviations and symbols

The purpose of punctuation is to make the written message easier to read and understand. To understand the importance of punctuation, read the following paragraph out loud:

> *Health-care professionals often work in teams a team that is committed to the task and makes full use of its members talents can achieve high levels of performance cooperation is needed for success in a spirit of cooperation people recognize the benefits of helping one another no one person has all the answers but each person has a piece of the puzzle once the pieces are shared the larger picture is clear and possible solutions are easier members need to feel important and that they have something to contribute they claim ownership when they have a share in making decisions carrying out policies or solving problems members must trust and have confidence in one another trust is built when there is an atmosphere of honesty fairness sensitivity and respect a trusting environment helps members to feel comfortable enough to share their talents and reveal their opinions people who benefit most from high quality performance are the patients*

The previous paragraph shows how difficult it is to make sense out of a text when punctuation is missing. Knowing how to use punctuation correctly is a crucial skill, especially for medical assistants. Doctors who dictate information often do not include punctuation. Punctuation makes sentences clearer, and good writing requires it.

Punctuation

The period, question mark, and exclamation point are referred to as end punctuation because they come at the ends of sentences. They mark the end of a complete thought.

The Period

A period is used at the end of a declarative sentence that makes a statement. A period is also used at the end of an imperative sentence that gives a command. In both cases, think about the period as a stop sign.

Examples

Bradycardia indicates a low pulse.

Prepare the patient for a gastrointestinal (GI) exam.

Follow the doctor's orders.

Schedule an appointment for next week.

Other Uses for the Period

Use a period to separate dollars and cents and whole numbers with decimals (decimal point). Do not use a period after whole numbers not accompanied by decimal fractions.

Examples

$6.50　*3.50 mm*　*0.43 cm*　*$25* (not *$25.00)*

1290　*16*　*21*

Use a period after most abbreviations.

Examples

Mr.　*Mrs.*　*Ms.*　*Rev.*　*Sr.*　*Dr.*　*B.S.*　*B.A.*　*M.S.*

M.Ed.　*Ph.D.*　*Esq.*　*John F. Smith*　*J.F. Smith*　*Jr.*

a.m.　*St.*　*Co.*　*Corp.*

Medically related abbreviations may appear in upper or lower case and with or without a period. Do not use periods with measurements.

Examples

i.e.　*etc.*　*et al.*　*cf.*　*b.i.d.*　*a.c.*　*h.s.*

mm　*cm*　*kg*　*ml*　*l*　*gl*　*mcg*　*mg*　*oz*　*ft*

A period is not placed after state abbreviations, zip codes, or acronyms. Acronyms are made up of the first letters in a series of words. They are sometimes pronounced as words.

Examples

Boston, *MA*　*OH*　*CT*　*FL*　*CA*　Douglas, *MA 01516*

AMA　*AAMA*　*CABG*　*AARP*　*OSHA*　*SIDS*

A period follows the letters and numbers in list or outline enumerations.

Examples

1. Nouns
2. Pronouns
3. Verbs

I. Medical Reports

A. History and Physical

B. Pathology

C. Discharge Summary

The Question Mark

A question mark is used after a direct question.

Examples

Where is the pain?

What is the diagnosis?

How much medication was ordered?

Do you know what the cure is for that disease?

"When can I go home?" asked the patient.

The Exclamation Point

Use the exclamation point after a sentence that expresses strong feelings.

Examples

Ouch! *Call security!*

CPR STAT! *Congratulations!*

What a wonderful way to stay healthy!

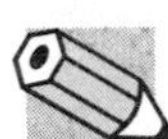

Practice 9-1

Place the appropriate punctuation marks at the ends of these sentences:

1. The trachea functions as a passageway for air to reach the lungs
2. Underage drinking is the largest drug problem in America
3. Is pruritus recorded as an objective symptom
4. The portion of the H&P where the physician uses hands and fingers during an examination is called palpation
5. Drinking kills 6.5 times as many children and teenagers than all other drugs combined
6. Is a curette used for scraping
7. Listening to sounds within the body is called auscultation
8. Bravo, we made our goal
9. Tapping the body for signs of disease is called percussion
10. STAT

The Comma

Within sentences, the comma is the most frequently used punctuation mark. It is also the punctuation mark that causes the most difficulty. Errors fall into two extreme categories: Commas are either disregarded or they are used too frequently. The main purpose of the comma is to group words that belong together and separate words that do not. A comma also represents a brief pause when reading. The best rule to follow about commas is not to use it unless there is a reason to do so.

Rule 1: The comma is used to separate three or more items in a series.

Examples

Coryza, cough, and sore throat are common in the winter.

Influenza is characterized by the sudden onset of *chills, headache, and myalgia.*

The five stages of grieving are *denial, anger, bargaining, depression, and acceptance.*

If items in a series are each linked by *and* or *or*, a comma is not used.

Examples

The four blood types are A *and* B *and* AB *and* O.

You could give 10 mg *or* 20 mg *or* 40 mg of Demerol I.M. for the pain.

Rule 2: Use a comma to separate two or more adjectives that describe the same noun.

Examples

Purulent, rusty-colored sputum was taken to the lab for testing.

The x-ray revealed *numerous, questionable nodules.*

Rule 3: A comma is used between two independent clauses joined by coordinating conjunctions (*and, but, or, not, for, so, yet*).

Examples

Medicare is administered by the Social Security Administration, *but the public welfare office handles Medicaid.*

Patients usually recover rapidly from influenza, *yet some patients experience lassitude for weeks.*

Did you hear about the new medication for arthritis, *and how it affects the elderly?*

Rule 4: Place a comma between the day and year. If a date is used in a sentence, a comma goes between the year and the rest of the sentence.

Examples

February 28, 2009

On *February 28, 2009*, the hospital will review its policies.

Rule 5: Use a comma between the city and state. When the city and state are used in a sentence, a comma is placed after the state.

Examples

Boston, Massachusetts

Anesthesia was first discovered in *Boston, Massachusetts,* at Massachusetts General Hospital.

The American Association of Medical Assistants and the American Medical Associations are located in *Chicago, IL.*

Rule 6: Use a comma to separate numbers that have four or more digits.

3,000 *30,000* *300,000* *3,000,000*

Exceptions include addresses and year numbers of four digits.

The address is *3600* Main Street.

Rule 7: Use a comma to separate appositives, nouns of direct address, titles that follow a person's name, and introductory words from the rest of the sentence.

Examples

Doctor, please listen carefully to what I have to say.

Please listen carefully, *Doctor,* to what I have to say.

Yes, you may have a regular diet.

However, I do think you will have to curtail your intake of cholesterol.

A decrease in total dietary fat will help, *however.*

Dr. Villes, *a pathologist,* graduated from a medical school in Burlington, VT.

The pathologist, *Norm Villes, M.D.,* graduated from a medical school in Burlington, VT.

Rule 8: Use a comma to separate clauses and phrases that are unnecessary to the meaning of a sentence (nonessential, or nonrestrictive, clauses and phrases).

Examples

The hospital, *unlike most facilities,* has a comprehensive evacuation plan. [*Unlike most facilities* is not necessary to the meaning of the sentence.]

The hourly pay, *in some circumstances,* increases over a period of time. [The sentence still makes sense when *in some circumstances* is omitted.]

Programs, *which are available on request*, are free of charge.

The healing was satisfactory, *treated with antibiotics.*

Rule 9: A comma follows the salutation in a friendly letter and the complementary close.

Examples

Yours truly, *Sincerely,* *Best regards,*

Dear Friend, *Hello, Bill,*

Rule 10: Separate parenthetical expressions with a comma, depending on where they are placed in the sentence. Parenthetical expressions include

I believe (think, hope, see, etc.)		*I am sure*	*on the contrary*
on the other hand	*after all*	*by the way*	*incidentally*
in fact	*indeed*	*naturally*	*of course*
in my opinion	*for example*	*however*	*nonetheless*
to tell the truth			

Examples

The surgery was successful. *Therefore,* there is no need of further treatment.

The report, *I hope*, will give you many options about treatments.

In my opinion, the signs and symptoms are indicative of angina pectoris.

An inadequate supply of oxygen to the myocardium, *for example*, is caused by arteriosclerosis.

Rule 11: Use a comma to separate a direct quotation.

Examples

The doctor said, "*You must give up smoking.*"

"*I really don't have the courage,*" the patient replied.

"*In that case,*" the doctor continued, "*you sign your own death warrant.*"

Rule 12: A comma is used to set off contrasting statements that are introduced by the words *not, rather,* and *though.*

Examples

Right now, *rather* than later, increase the medication.

I would describe her mood as thoughtful, *not* sullen.

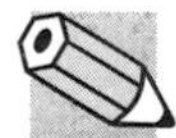

Practice 9-2

Punctuate these sentences:

1. The divisions of the vertebrae are cervical thoracic lumbar sacral and coccygeal
2. Combining forms prefixes and suffixes are used to build medical words
3. The computer program includes the software
4. Medical histories are entered into a file on a word processor
5. A tickler file is a reference system of call-back appointment dates and future events
6. On the other hand correspondence relating to administration is filed by subject

7. Demographic information includes the date of birth place of residence and insurance

8. After she read the lab reports she called the resident

9. Prior to antibiotics her sinusitis caused headaches

10. The symptoms are vomiting drowsiness shock pallor diaphoresis and liver tenderness

11. The patient with the CABG needs blood work

12. The patient is instructed to wash the skin avoid scrubbing and keep hands away from the face

13. Would you please hand me the towel nurse

14. I don't believe it

15. If one side is normal and the other is not a comparison between the two may be made

16. The patient replied "I don't want my family to know"

17. The administration after all is also responsible for what happens in the hospital

18. Is there a history of myocardial infarctions in the family

19. After July 15 send my mail to Albany NY 02863

20. All must attend the meeting be on time and participate

21. At night it is a swollen painful joint

22. Symptoms appeared six weeks after the primary lesion occurred principally on the mucous membranes

23. Deterioration of arterial blood gases increased the patient's breathing efforts decreased his energy and put him in an unstable condition

24. Two famous women in medicine by the way are Florence Nightingale and Clara Barton

25. Louis Pasteur a Frenchman did brilliant work in chemistry and bacteriology and is one of the most famous men in medical history

26. In 1928 Sir Alexander Fleming discovered penicillin

27. Who is the person responsible for x-ray therapy

28. A pathological condition of the body exhibits signs and symptoms of a disease

29. After a period of time syphilis can cause blindness insanity heart disease and death

30. Pain suffering and stress from illnesses are different with each individual

The Semicolon

The semicolon is a punctuation mark that is stronger than a comma; that is, it indicates a more definite break in the flow of a sentence. Semicolons join items that are grammatically alike or closely related.

Rule 1: A semicolon is used instead of a comma and a coordinating conjunction (*and, but, or, nor, for, yet* and *so*) to separate two independent clauses.

Examples

A physician shall respect the law; recognize the responsibility to change any law that is contrary to the best interest of the patient.

Almost all victims of violence go to emergency centers; many have no health insurance.

Many people are homeless because they were discharged from a mental institution; most are without proper follow-up health care.

If a coordinating conjunction is present, commas are used to separate independent clauses. The clauses can also be rewritten as two sentences.

Examples

The cost of health care in the U.S. is out of control; 37 million have no health insurance and 35 million are underinsured.

The cost of health care in the U.S. is out of control, yet 37 million have no health insurance and 35 million are underinsured.

The cost health care in the U. S. is out of control. Thirty-seven million have no health insurance and thirty-five million are underinsured.

Rule 2: Use a semicolon between independent clauses when the second clause begins with a transitional expression such as:

for example	*for instance*	*otherwise*
that is	*besides*	*therefore*
accordingly	*moreover*	*consequently*
nevertheless	*furthermore*	*however*
instead	*hence*	*namely*

Examples

Every medical office has its unique pathology format; *however*, the data required is the same.

The arterial blood gas reports are good; *therefore*, we can begin the process of weaning from the ventilator.

The cardiac rate was rapid and regular; *consequently*, there are no extrasystoles.

The patient was afebrile after admission; *nevertheless*, he became febrile with recurrent episodes of pain in the left side of the chest.

Note: A comma sets off one independent clause: "*The medical report is completed,* all ten pages." A semicolon sets off two independent clauses: "The medical report is completed; mail it first class."

Rule 3: Use a semicolon with a series of items that have one or more commas.

Examples

Those present at the meeting were Dr. M. P. Carr, my family physician; Mrs. P. Archy, my lawyer; Bob, my husband; and Valerie, my daughter.

I sent copies to Burlington, Vermont; Concord, New Hampshire; and Boston, Massachusetts.

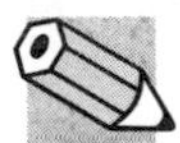

Practice 9-3

Punctuate these sentences:

1. I wanted a response from Dr. Ville a forensic pathologist from Boston but as of today I received none
2. Call Dr. Sarah the surgeon Kim Yonta the lawyer and Chris Ville the medical insurance representative
3. Val visited the medical library on Tuesday she also did further research on Saturday
4. The importance of determining the comparability of the two drug groups is evident for example eleven deaths to surgery five to acute myocardial infarction and six to embolic complications
5. Soon redness pain and swelling appeared in the right ankle consequently ice packs were applied

The Colon

The colon is a sign that more information follows. The information may be expressed in a series of words, phrases, or clauses.

Rule 1: A colon is used to introduce a list or series of items.

Examples

The pathology report consists of the following: the patient's name, medical record number, tissues submitted, findings, impressions, and possible treatment.

The only explanations I can give are these: the patient didn't follow directions, forgot to take the medication, or stopped taking it because of side effects.

I made a list of the things we need: forceps, 4-0 catgut sutures, gauze sponges, and surgical scissors.

I made a list of the things we need:

1. forceps
2. 4-0 catgut sutures
3. gauze sponges
4. surgical scissors

Rule 2: A colon is not used if a verb or preposition immediately precedes series of the items. Whatever precedes a colon should be a complete sentence.

Examples

The health team consists *of* physicians, nurses, a physical therapist, and a nurse aide. [preposition]

We *need* forceps, 4-0 catgut sutures, gauze sponges, and suture scissors. [verb]

Rule 3: A colon is used between hours and minutes to express time.

6:15 8:30 a.m. 8 a.m. (Do not use zeros for on-the-hour time.)

Rule 4: A colon is used in business letters.

Examples

Dear Dr. Villes:

To Whom It May Concern:

Re: Medical Report #1234235

CC: President Vernon
Valerie Christopher

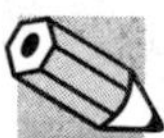

Practice 9-4

Punctuate these sentences:

1. SOCIAL HISTORY The patient neither smokes nor drinks
2. Is my appointment at 11 30 or 1 30
3. Many medical assistants were at the Cancer Conference Chris Luke John Valerie and Sarah
4. Tissues involved

   1 Node from the left lung

   2 Right mediastinal nodes

3 Carina

4 Left lung

5. Discharge diagnoses

A Excision of benign cyst of left lung

B Emphysema

C Klebsiella pneumoniae infection

6. Fibrous tissue extending out from the vitreous was covered with many vessels

7. To Whom It May Concern

8. Digitalis therapy was begun because of dyspnea chest pain and swelling of the legs

9. The cases were arterial insufficiency diabetes gangrene glomerulonephritis and anemia

10. Marked interstitial edema was present with diffuse mononuclear infiltrate composed of lymphocytes and plasma

Parentheses

Rule 1: Parentheses surround information that is added but unnecessary and unrelated to the main thought of the sentence.

Example

The nurses from the second floor *(Lisa, Kurt, Nancy, and Ramon)* make a great team.

Rule 2: Parentheses are used a round an abbreviation or acronym that follows the spelled out version, or vice versa.

Examples

The medical assistant *(M.A.)* is responsible for typing the report.

OSHA *(Occupational Health and Safety Association)* provides valuation information to hospitals.

Rule 3: Use parentheses around numerals or italic letters that designate enumerations of list items within a sentence.

Examples

The instructions are *(a)* more fluids, *(b)* A.S.A. 2 tabs prn, and *(c)* bedrest.

The instructions are (1) more fluids, (2) A.S.A. 2 tabs prn, and (3) bedrest.

The Dash

The purpose of the dash (—) is to set off unnecessary items from the rest of the sentence. The reason for using the dash, rather than any other punctuation mark, is to give more emphasis to words. The dash may be applied singly or in pairs. However, it is rarely seen in medical documentation.

Examples

I have 30 years—*very rewarding ones*—of medical practice.

The forms are to be written exclusively by physicians—*not nurses, not therapists, not social workers, and not aides.*

The Hyphen

The hyphen was covered in Chapter 4, under "Predicate and Compound Adjectives." Because punctuation is so important in medical documentation, a short review is included here.

Rule 1: Use a hyphen between compound words used as an adjective when the adjective precedes the noun.

Examples

all-day surgery   *102-year-old* man   *grayish-black* tissue

follow-up   *one-by-one*

A *well-developed, well-nourished* young man.

A *34-year-old* male was admitted to the West Wing.

When a compound word follows the noun, it is not hyphenated.

The young man was *well developed.*

Compound words that have become commonly used are not hyphenated.

earache   *gallbladder*   *nosebleed*

Rule 2: Use a hyphen with numbers 21 to 99 and with written fractions.

thirty-five days ago   *one-third of the hospital rooms*

Rule 3: Use a hyphen with a prefix added to a word that begins with a capital letter.

mid-March   *un-American*

Rule 4: Some adjective forms are always hyphenated, whether before of after the nouns they modify.

self-conscious   *cross-referenced*

Rule 5: Use a hyphen in some compound words used as nouns.

mother-in-law *check-up* *work-up* *ex-employer*

Always consult the dictionary when in doubt about hyphenation.

The Apostrophe

Another punctuation mark often used in medical reporting is the apostrophe. An apostrophe is used to show ownership (referred to as the possessive form of a noun).

The apostrophe was covered in detail in Chapter 1 in Figure 1-5.

Italics

Italic print is used for emphasis, words used as terms, or words used as words. If italic print is not available, underlining is used.

Examples

All surgical equipment *must* be sterilized before use.

The term *officious* could be applied to his tone in the letter.

Friendly and *polite* are not synonymous.

Italics are also used in the following instances:

- Titles of books, magazines, and newspapers

  New England Journal of Medicine

  New York Times Gray's Anatomy

  Lancet *Taber's Cyclopedic Medical Dictionary*

  Harvard Health Letter *JAMA*

- Movies, television, radio, plays, and operas

  Mozart's Requiem

  Did you watch *ER* on television last night?

- Foreign expressions

  mea culpa: my fault

  fait accompli: carried out with success

  respondeat superior: "Let the master answer."

  res ipsa loquitur: "Let the thing speak for itself."

- All biological names

  Clostridium difficile Staphylococcus aureus

  Streptococcus pyogenes *Escherichia coli*

  Pseudomonas aeruginosa *Salmonella enteritidis*

  Haemophilus influenza *Campylobacter jejuni*

Quotation Marks

Quotation marks are used to enclose the exact words of the speaker. Quotations are often used in the subjective part of POMR charting, or when it is necessary to quote the exact words of the patient or a family member.

Examples

Robert said, "*I have pain in my chest.*" [The period goes inside the quotation mark when words apply only to the quoted material.]

"*I go to physical therapy at 3 p.m.,*" said Sheila. [Note the comma *inside* the quote.]

"*Take the patient to room 205,*" Robert said, "*while I bring the chart to the desk.*" [Note the interruption of the quotation.]

"*What was the FBS?*" asked Dr. Oberg. [Note the question mark *inside* the quote.]

"*I would advise caution,*" said the physician, "*because your condition is serious.*"

Quotation marks are also used to enclose a part of a completed published work or to indicate that words or phrases are being used in a special way.

Examples

Chapter 9 is titled "Punctuation."

The title of the seminar is "Stress Management."

Write "confidential" on the envelope.

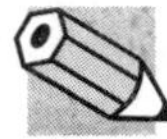

Practice 9-5

Punctuate these sentences:

1. The chapter entitled punctuation is the most important chapter in the book.
2. Quick said John get the defibrilator!
3. We got the article out the New England Journal of Medicine.
4. The vertebrae are composed of thirty three bony segments.
5. Yogurt is a form of curdled milk caused by Lactobacillus bulgaricus.
6. The preoperative medication is due forty five minutes before surgery.
7. The side effects of the medication are 1 headaches 2 possible vomiting and 3 diarrhea.
8. The speaker was very self conscious.
9. Yellow fever is caused by the bite of the female mosquito Aedes aegypti.
10. JAMA and the Lancet published the study.

Medical Spelling

Become familiar with the spelling of the following words:

afebrile
anesthesia
angina
arteriosclerosis
buccal
cholesterol
curette
defibrillator
digitalis
earache
embolus
febrile
filtration
forceps
hematology
infiltrate
insufficiency
interstitial
Kaposis' sarcoma
keratitis
myalgia
myocardium
neuromuscular
nodules
norepinephrine
opaque
papilla
penicillin
percussion
purulent
Salmonella
Staphylococcus
Streptococcus
tracheostomy
thrombus
ventilate
vitreous
well-developed
well-nourished
Xylocaine

Punctuation Study Summary

Period*

After a statement	You looked better after your treatments.
With abbreviations.	Dr. R. Williams. a.m. $50
Not with abbreviations of measurements	3.5 mm ft gal

Question Mark

After a question	At what time is the operation scheduled?
	How old were you on your last birthday?

Exclamation Point

After an exclamatory sentence	Your house is on fire!
	Get help in here right away!

*The period, question mark, and exclamation point are referred to as end punctuation because they come at the ends of sentences.

Comma: Used to group words that belong together, separate words that do not belong together, and provide a brief pause.

In a series	The recovery rooms are painted in aqua, light blue, lavendar, and white.
Between two adjectives before a noun	A confidant, trustworthy nurse is hard to find.
	I'm looking for an inexpensive, comfortable car.
Before *and, but, or, nor, yet* following an independent clause	I have good medical coverage, but it expires when I leave my job.
Around unnecessary clauses and phrases	Computers, used correctly, can save a lot of time. To the best of my knowledge, the situation no longer exists.
	Looking ahead, we can prepare for the event.
Following introductory elements	Well, we can do it again to make sure.
Around parenthetical expressions	In fact, I did pass with honors.
Around appositives	If you believe that, John, you can believe anything.
Other uses	
Following the salutation of a friendly letter	Dear Mom,
Following a complimentary close	Sincerely yours,
Between city and state	Chicago, Illinois 68594
Between date and year	October 11, 20XX
To separate quotations	"I drove by car," replied the salesman.
In numbers of four or more digits	600,000
Preceding a title after a person's name	Dr. William Borden, Ph.D.

Semicolon: Used to indicate a more definite break than a comma in the flow of a sentence and to join items that are grammatically alike or closely related.

Between independent clauses not joined by a coordinating conjunction (*and, but, or*)	I saw red; I was so angry.
Between independent clauses joined by *however, hence, that is, therefore,* etc.	Computers are faster; therefore, use them for scheduling appointments.
Separating elements in a series that contain commas	Cities and countries participating are Rome, Italy; London, England; and Ottawa, Canada.

Colon: Used to indicate that more information is coming.

Preceding a series, lists, or outlines that are not introduced by a verb.	Consider the following: less expensive, better quality, and good returns on investment.
Between minutes and hours in expressions of time	9:15 p.m.

Following the time salutation of a business letter	Dear Mr. President:

Parentheses ( ): Used to mark off explanations.

Around added information unrelated to the main thought	The physicians (all eight of them) donated services to the needy.
Around words added to clarify the sentence	The AMA (American Medical Association) is a powerful organization.
Around numbers or letters that designate enumerations of list items within a sentence	The best things to do are (1) take a fever reducer, (2) get plenty of rest, and (3) drink a lot of fluids.

Dash: Used to set off unnecessary items from the rest of the sentence.

Adds emphasis	She won the prize—a trip to Disney World.

Hyphen: Used between elements of compound words or numbers and to divide words into syllables.

Compound words, syllables	state-of-the-art equipment
	mu-sic
With written numbers 21 to 99	twenty-five years ago
In written fractions	one-half the population
Between a prefix and the base word	un-American
	self-explanatory

Apostrophe: Used to Show ownership.

Forms the possessive	Singular: patient's disease, boss's
	Plural: patients' disease, bosses'

Italics: Used in place of an underline to point out or emphasize.

For names of books, magazines, works of art, biological names, foreign expressions.	I subscribe to the *PMA*. *E. Coli* is normal flora in the G.I. tract.

Quotation marks: Used to enclose the exact words of a speaker.

Around a direct quote	The doctor said, "Be sure to take your medication."
Around all segments of an interrupted quote	"Be sure to take your medicine," said the doctor, "or you won't get well."
Around parts of published works	The article "The Pathology of Germs" can be found on the Internet.
Around words or phrases used in a special way	The president's diagnosis was so "confidential" that even reporters were aware of it.

Skills Review

Punctuate these sentences:

1. Soft relaxing music is soothing to patients waiting in a doctor office
2. Because new drugs are pure chemicals they are dispensed by weight
3. Four common routes of antibiotic are intravenous intramuscular oral and local
4. By the way on November 7 2002 my cast will be taken off
5. If you do not receive your raise by the first of the year be sure to inform the personnel department
6. Objects should never be placed inside a cast to relieve itching relief comes by applying a cold pack over the cast where the itch is located
7. A patient is instructed on how to care for the cast limit activities use devices such as crutches or a cane and perform prescribed exercises
8. Stages of a cataract are 1 cloudlike opacities 2 swollen lens 3 opaque lens and 4 solid or shrunken lens
9. After a period of time syphilis can cause blindness insanity heart disease and death
10. Coryza is a general term for a cold or inflammation of the respiratory mucous membranes
11. OTC mediations are available for cough headache and fever
12. The large intestines are about 1.5 mm long and are divided into 4 parts the ascending the transverse the descending and the sigmoid colon
13. The Fairfield Medical Center where the surgery takes place has an excellent staff of surgeons
14. The patient I hope will sign the Release of Information form
15. The sales representative covers the cities of Worcester MA Providence RI and Hartford CT
16. By combining prefixes and suffixes new medical words are formed
17. Diabetes meaning passing through is a general term for excessive urination and is usually referred to as diabetes mellitus
18. Those present were Dr Saggot the cardiologist Dr Dermody the hematologist and Dr Downs the endocrinologist

19. Three CMAs are on call this weekend Ms Zimmerman Ms Perez and Mr Weinhart

20. Special stains display the evidence of acid fast bacilli within the granulomata

21. ADMITTING DIAGNOSIS Rule out cholecystitis cholelithiasis

22. LABORATORY DATA Sodium 140 potassium 3.0 chloride 100 SGOT 40 and SGPT 34

23. ALLERGIES None known

24. This is a 34 year old white male

25. Gentlemen

26. HEENT normocephalic NECK supple HEART without gallops or murmurs

27. Come in at 1015 a m

28. Complete straight leg raises to 45 degrees q i d

29. The specimen consists of a gallbladder measuring 7.8 × 4 cm

30. If any problems develop such as the following fever nausea vomiting headaches or blurred vision come to the emergency room

Circle the correct spelling word in each line.

1. ceratitis	keratitis	karatitis	kerratitis
2. kolesterol	cholisterol	cholesterol	cholestirol
3. interstitiol	interstichial	interstiel	interstitial
4. myalgia	mialgia	myalgea	myolgia
5. artiriosclerosis	arteriscelrosis	arteriosclerosis	arterioclerosis
6. Strepcoccus	Stretcocucus	Steptococcus	Streptococcus
7. bukkal	bucal	buccal	buccle
8. insuficiency	insufficiency	insifficency	insphiciency
9. Xylocaine	Xylocane	Xylicaine	Zylocaine
10. pencillin	penicillin	penecillin	pinicilin

Punctuate and capitalize these sentences:

Health care professionals often work in teams a team committed to the task makes full use of its members talents and can achieve high levels of performance cooperation is needed for success in a spirit of cooperation people recognize the benefits of helping one another no one person has all the answers but each person has a piece of the puzzle once the pieces are shared the larger picture is clear and possible solutions are easier members need to feel important and that they have something to contribute they claim ownership when they have a share in making decisions carrying out policies or solving problems members must trust and have confidence in one another trust is built when there is an atmosphere of honesty fairness sensitivity and respect a trusting environment helps members to feel comfortable enough to share their talents and reveal their opinions people who benefit most from high quality performance are the patients.

Translate these medical abbreviations using a medical dictionary or appendix.

1. ung. ____________________
2. TIA ____________________
3. T&A ____________________
4. S/P ____________________
5. TMJ ____________________
6. t/o ____________________
7. ≈ ____________________
8. tinct ____________________
9. UE ____________________
10. + ____________________

Chapter 10

The Paragraph

Objectives

Upon completion of this chapter, the student should be able to:

- recognize and write different types of paragraphs
- understand the structure and development of a paragraph
- organize and compose paragraphs according to various approaches to sentence progression
- use various techniques to attain paragraph unity
- spell various medical terms
- translate various medical abbreviations and symbols

Chapter 8 shows how individual parts of speech are arranged to form a coherent sentence. This chapter explains how sentences are joined together to form a coherent paragraph. A paragraph is a group of sentences that go together because they explain a common point of view called a *main idea.* A main idea is the central message that the writer wishes to convey to the reader. That message is what drives the entire passage. Every sentence in an effective paragraph must be related to the main idea.

A paragraph is easy to detect because the start of its first sentence is indented about five spaces from the left-hand margin. The length of a paragraph varies, depending on the complexity of the main idea. The average length of an effective paragraph ranges from four to eight sentences. Readers lose their focus when a paragraph is too long or too short. In medical documentation, paragraphs differ in length, depending on the amount of medical facts included in them.

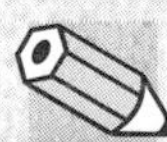

Practice 10-1

All three of the following paragraphs give the same message. Which one is easier to read and understand?

1. The doctor's office is more than a professional health-care service. It is also a business. Because of this reality, an efficient system of record management is needed to maintain a well-directed medical office practice. The first component of medical records deals with a patient's health information. Data include such items as a medical history, examination results, record of treatments, laboratory reports, prescriptions, and diagnoses. Invoices, insurance forms and policies, payroll records, canceled checks, financial records, and other correspondence pertain to the business component of the operation. More than likely, business information is filed separately from a patient's health record. Medical professionals may draw on four or five different filing methods to maintain order: alphabetic, numeric, geographic, subject, and color-coding. Efficient record management is essential for the smooth operation of both components of a medical office practice.

2. The doctor's office is more than a professional health-care service. It is also a business. - Because of this reality, an efficient system of record management is needed to maintain a well-directed medical office practice.

The first component of medical records deals with a patient's health information. Data include such items as a medical history, examination results, record of treatments, laboratory reports, prescriptions, and diagnoses. Invoices, insurance forms and policies, payroll records, canceled checks, financial records, and other general correspondence pertain to the business component of the operation.

More than likely, business information is filed separately from a patient's health record. Medical professionals may draw on four or five different filing methods to maintain order: alphabetic, numeric, geographic, subject, and color-coding. Efficient record management is essential for the smooth operation of both segments of a medical office practice.

3. The doctor's office is more than a professional health-care service. It is also a business. Because of this reality, an efficient system of record management is needed to maintain a well-directed medical office practice.

The first component of medical records deals with a patient's health information.

Data include such items as a medical history, examination results, record of treatments, laboratory reports, prescriptions, and diagnoses.

Invoices, insurance forms and policies, payroll records, canceled checks, financial records, and other general correspondence pertain to the business component of the operation.

More than likely, business information is filed separately from a patient's health report.

Medical professionals may draw on four or five different filing methods to maintain order: alphabetic, numeric, geographic, subject, and color-coding.

Efficient record management is essential for the smooth operation of both components of a medical office practice.

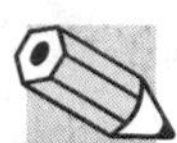

Practice 10-2

Separate this short essay into three paragraphs:

Patients often wonder why the social history (SH) component is part of medical records. On further investigation into the meaning of social history, the reason becomes evident. Habits of smoking, physical exercises, eating, sleeping, and hobbies greatly impact the health of every individual. Facts about a patient's family history provide the physician with additional health data. Hereditary factors, and parent and sibling health conditions help doctors see the larger picture. Questions on the review of symptoms (ROS) concentrate on the patient's general health condition unrelated to the present illness. The ROS provides a history of systems and organs, usually in logical order from head to foot.

____

____

____

____

____

____

____

Types of Paragraphs

Many different types of paragraphs exist. The four types most commonly encountered by people in the medical profession are narrative, descriptive, expository, and persuasive.

Narrative Paragraph

As the word implies, a narrative paragraph describes a story or a series of events that usually occur in chronological order. Narrative paragraphs may be autobiographical (about oneself) or biographical (about another), or about something witnessed.

Example

Elizabeth Blackwell, an immigrant from England, was the first woman in the U.S. to receive a degree in medicine. She was refused entrance into medical school many times before she was finally accepted. While practicing in this country, she established a hospital staffed by women. Returning to England, she founded the London School of Medicine for Women.

Descriptive Paragraph

A descriptive paragraph is a pictorial representation in words of the sort that appears in most types of writing. The choice of words in this type of paragraph is deliberately specific to describe concrete details about objects, ideas, actions, settings, or persons. The wording conveys a sensory impression of smell, taste, sound, touch or reveals a mood or an emotion.

Example

The professor in the anatomy lab described the heart in the following manner:

The heart is a muscular organ located between the lungs. It weighs about nine ounces and is about the size of a fist. The heart has four chambers. The two upper chambers, the atria, are the receiving chambers and the two lower chambers, the ventricles, are the pumping chambers. Valves are located between the upper and lower chambers that open and close to let the flow of blood pass in one direction.

Expository Paragraph

An expository paragraph is the most common type of paragraph. Its purpose is to inform, explain, or define something. The information may include facts, statistics, or specific examples. Because the language is so precise, the tone of the paragraph is very factual and unemotional.

Example

The patient's chief complaint is headache pain on one side of the head. If this is a migraine, it exhibits certain characteristics, Migraines have a high hereditary influence and commonly affect more women than men. The usual symptoms are severe, intense, and of long duration. It often presents when the person wakes in the morning. One side of the head is affected more than the other. The pain may be more severe over the temporal area, but also may include the face and other areas of the head. Other signs and symptoms that may occur at the attack are nausea and/or vomiting, fatigue, irritability, chilliness, edema, diaphoresis, or aphasia.

Persuasive Paragraph

The persuasive paragraph is written to urge the reader to follow a certain course of action, to deal with an important issue, or to state an opinion about a debatable issue. The topic sentence clearly and concisely states the writer's point of view. Subsequent sentences develop the issue with reasonable and supportive statements.

Example

One critical pathway for increasing the effectiveness of medical care in hospitals is to adopt quality assurance standards. These standards encompass every facet of the hospital; from medical personnel, patients, staff, and administration. Other components include medical care, patients' rights, family satisfaction, hospital policies, cost-effectiveness, and medical records. The Joint Commission on Accreditation of Healthcare Organizations establishes quality assurance standards. The implementation of these standards is a necessity if growth is to take place in the health care industry.

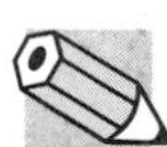

Practice 10-3

Identify this paragraph as descriptive, exclamatory, or persuasive:

Electrolytes are chemical compounds found in all body fluids. Electrolytes break into positive and negative particles that conduct electrical impulses. Acids, bases, and salts are examples of electrolytes. Some general functions of all electrolytes are: (1) to promote neuromuscular irritability, (2) to maintain body fluid volume, (3) to distribute water between fluid compartments, and (4) to help regulate the acid-base balance. Electrolytes are a necessity for life.

Structure of a Paragraph

The structure of the paragraph consists of three elements: the topic sentence, supporting sentences, and a concluding sentence. The topic sentence presents the main idea. Subsequent supporting sentences offer more details about the topic. The concluding sentence brings closure to the paragraph (Figure 10-1).

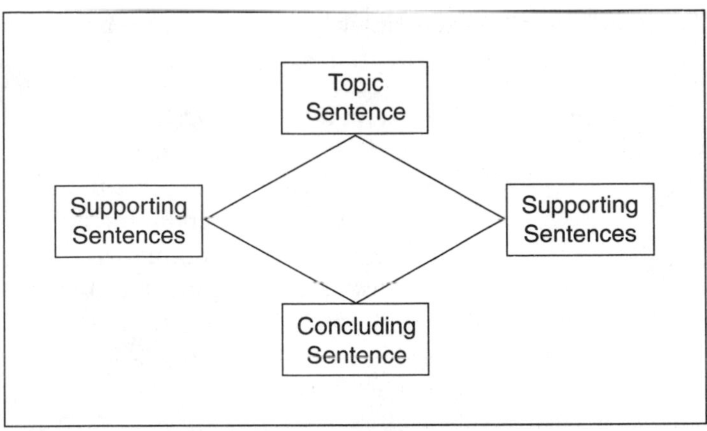

Figure 10-1 The structure of an effective paragraph

Topic Sentence

The topic sentence is the most important sentence in the paragraph because it introduces the reader to the main idea. It tells the reader what the paragraph is about and helps keep ideas organized and focused. In a sense, the paragraph is a clear and direct summary of the main idea. A paragraph without a topic sentence misdirects and confuses the reader. The topic sentence should immediately capture the interest of the reader.

Supporting Sentences

The supporting sentences form the body of the paragraph and comprise the details, facts, examples, descriptions, definitions, explanations, questions, causes and effects, comparisons, contrasts, and proofs that support the main idea expressed in the topic sentence. The more specific the details of the supporting sentences, the better the explanation of the main idea. The content of the body usually answers any number of questions like *who? what? what kind? where? when? why?* and *how?*

Concluding Sentence

The final sentence brings the paragraph to a conclusion in one of several ways. It may summarize, offer a solution, predict, make a recommendation, state a conclusion, or restate the topic sentence.

Putting It All Together

Example 1

Topic Sentence	Punctuation is a crucial skill for medical assistants to possess.
Supporting Sentences	Many physicians do not bother to punctuate their reports, letters, notes, or correspondence. Should punctuation be included, it is oftentimes used incorrectly. The end punctuation of sentences is usually correct because the punctuation marks are obvious. The punctuation mark that causes the most problems, however, is the comma. There are more rules for the use of the comma than any other type of punctuation.

Concluding Sentence	Knowing where to place commas is a crucial step in acquiring punctuation skills.
The Complete Paragraph	Punctuation is a crucial skill for medical assistants to possess. Many physicians do not bother to punctuate their letters, notes, or correspondence. Should punctuation be included, it is oftentimes used incorrectly. The end punctuation of sentences is usually correct because the punctuation marks are obvious. The punctuation mark that causes the most problems, however, is the comma. There are more rules for the use of the comma than any other type of punctuation. Knowing where to place commas is a crucial step in acquiring punctuation skills.

Example 2

Topic Sentence	An operative note is one type of medical documentation.
Supporting Sentences	This report describes a surgical operation, dictated by the surgeon or an assistant. The report includes pre- and postoperative diagnoses, sponge count, and blood loss.
Concluding Sentence	The report concludes with the patient's condition at the end of the surgical procedure.
The Complete Paragraph	An operative note is one type of medical documentation. The report describes a surgical operation, dictated by the surgeon or an assistant. The report includes pre- and postoperative diagnoses, sponge count, and blood loss. The report concludes with the patient's condition at the end of the surgical procedure.

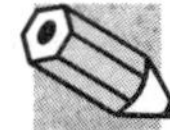

Practice 10-4

Identify the topic, supporting, and concluding sentences in each paragraph:

1. The rate of respiration may be normal, rapid, or slow. The average rate for an adult is 12 to 20 cycles per minute. The average for infants is 30 to 60. For children age one to seven, the rate is 18 to 30 cycles per minute. The number per minute is referred to as the rate of respiration. Medical office workers should be aware of these facts.

2. Gerontology is the study of the aging process. During this process, the chemical composition of the body changes. Among these changes are a decrease in lean body mass and an increase in vulnerability to different diseases. Stress is also an important factor in aging. Stress decreases cardiac output and brain function. As a result, the aging population is more susceptible to infections and accidents.

3. The electrocardiogram (EKG or ECG) is a recorded picture of the electrical activity of the heart. The EKG may be normal even in the presence of heart disease. It is essential that the EKG be used in conjunction with the patient history, physical exam, and laboratory data. Arrhythmia and dysrhythmia are used interchangeably to denote an abnormal conduction. Electrocardiograms are a necessary component in assessing cardiovascular disease.

4. Communication consists of many types. The spoken word or verbal communication is not the only one. Sometimes people communicate more with actions than with

words. A smile or frown, eye contact or lack of it, gestures, postures, touch, and style of dress are expressions of nonverbal communication. In these cases, actions may speak louder than words.

5. Fats, proteins, carbohydrates, vitamins, and minerals are all necessary nutrients for the body. A person's basal metabolic rate, growth, and physical activity determine the amount of nutrients needed. Nutrition needs change when a person is ill, is taking medications, or has a type of trauma. An imbalance occurs when nutrients are consumed in concentrated forms and reach the point that they do not help. Proper nutrition is important to everyone's health.

Paragraph Organization

Paragraphs should be well organized in that the arrangement of their sentences should follow some order. Two common ways to organize paragraphs are by time and logic. Time is a chronological approach that lists events from the earliest to the most recent, or in reverse, from the most recent to the earliest. An example of time is a paragraph describing events from 1989 to 2010; a resume is an example of reverse chronological order. Organization by time is commonly used for paragraphs telling about experiences or actions, for biographical paragraphs, or for historical accounts.

Time Example

The AMA was organized in 1846 in New York City. A Code of Ethics was formulated and adopted in 1847. Its principles were revised in 1906, 1912, and 1949. In 1957, they were condensed to a preamble and ten sections.

Organizing paragraphs by time, however, is not conducive to documenting ideas. To write about ideas, paragraphs are organized by logic. Paragraphs organized by logic proceed from the familiar to the less familiar, simple points to more complex points, less important things to more important things, and the general to the specific.

Logic Example

Treason is a crime against a nation. Major crimes like robbery, arson, and forgery are felonies. Misdemeanors are lesser crimes. An example of an misdemeanor in the medical profession is possession of an unauthorized hypodermic needle. An infraction is a minor offense that results in a fine.

Other ways to organize paragraphs are location, deduction, induction, cause and effect, comparison, and definition or classification. The location approach involves the arrangement of content from left to right, right to left, top to bottom, edge to center, and the like.

Location Example

Chart notes are dictated in a SOAP format. *S* refers to *subjective* or what the patient tells the doctor. The *O* for *objective* consists of what the physician finds on examination. *A* is the *assessment* the physician makes or the diagnosis. *P* stands for the *planned* course of treatment.

Organizing by deduction starts with the general and goes to the specific. The topic sentence, which is general, is followed with specific reasons, examples, facts, and details that support the topic sentence.

Deduction Example

Follow these general rules regarding word contractions in medical transcription. Contractions may be used in informal records like chart notes. However, in formal correspondence like reports, use the words that form the contraction (do not, is not) rather than the contractions (don't, isn't).

Induction is the opposite of deduction. Specific ideas come before the general. Details, reasons, and examples follow the topic sentence.

Induction Example

Letters to insurance companies and physicians are a few examples of correspondence dictated by specialists. To this list may be added follow-up letters concerning referred patients and letters of introduction. Medical office correspondence consists of many different types.

Cause and effect paragraphs help connect the result of something with the events or facts that precede it.

Cause and Effect Example

Prilosec stops the production of stomach acid. It can turn off stomach acid production within an hour. The medication is used for conditions in which stomach acid is produced as part of a condition. Some of the drug's side effects are headache, diarrhea, nausea, fever, and vomiting.

The comparison paragraph measures one subject against another subject. The comparison is presented early. Contrasted details are given to illustrate the differences between the subjects.

Comparison Example

Legal abuses that affect health care are physical abuse and verbal abuse. Examples of physical abuse are performing the wrong treatment, hitting, holding the patient too roughly, or failing to answer the call light. Verbal abuse is using profanity or raising a voice in anger. Failure to obey laws regarding abuse results in fines or imprisonment.

Paragraphs organized by definition or classification paragraphs explain words and ideas in a clear fashion.

Definition Example

Pulse, respiration, temperature, and blood pressure are called vital signs. Pulse is the regular throbbing of the arteries echoing contractions of the heart. Respiration is the process of breathing and is measured by watching a patient breath in and out. Temperature is the degree of heat within the body. Blood pressure is the amount of force exerted by the heart pumping blood though the arteries. Vital signs are extremely important because appropriate medical care depends on these readings.

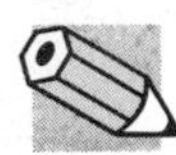

Practice 10-5

Identify the following paragraphs as organized by time, logic, induction, cause and effect, comparison, location, deduction, definition, or classification:

1. *Advice* is a noun that means an opinion or a recommendation: My *advice* to you is to get a second opinion. *Advise* is a verb that means to inform or to recommend: I would *advise* you to get a second opinion. ________________

2. When arranging flight reservations for the medical conference, obtain departure date and time, flight number, and estimated time of arrival. Make hotel reservations and arrange transportation from the airport to the hotel in time for the conference. The same information is required for the return trip: transportation to the airport, departure and arrival times, and arrangements to be picked up at the airport and driven home. ________________

3. Alzheimer's disease is caused by changes in nerve endings and brain cells that interfere with normal brain function. Symptoms of Alzheimer's progress from simple forgetfulness to severe loss of memory on how to dress, eat, or call people by name. Other signs are unpredictable moods and personality changes. ________________

4. *Effect* is a noun that means the result of some action: The side *effect* of antihistamine may make you sleepy. *Affect* is usually a verb that means to impress or influence, usually in the mind or feelings: The death of the patient *affected* us. ________________

5. Locating a file on the computer is likened to locating a file in a file cabinet. Entering the A or C drive on the computer is similar to opening a drawer of the file cabinet. Clicking the subdirectory on the computer (A:Dr. Villes/consults) is comparable to opening a file pulled from the drawer. ________________

Paragraph Unity

In addition to structure and organization, an effective paragraph should also have unity. Unity means that sentences should flow logically from one statement to another. Ideas are arranged and connected so they will read smoothly and sensibly. Paragraph unity is achieved in a number of ways, one of which is called *transition.* A transition is a word, phrase, or structural element that appropriately links one sentence to the next by referring to previously used words or ideas:

> *Bathing* is as important to the sick as it is to persons who are well. *Besides* removing dirt and perspiration, *bathing* helps patients relax.

Examples of transitional words are *finally, consequently, also, thus, in another sense, in the same way, specifically, nevertheless, nonetheless, besides, on the other hand, above, below, meanwhile, moreover, however, as I said above, still, therefore, furthermore, in addition, similarly, in contrast, on the contrary, for example, accordingly, as a result, consequently, next, finally, yet, that is, in particular, at last, likewise, more important, then, in summary, on the whole, as a matter of fact, during, after, before,* and *the first point.*

Transitional words can be grouped by location, time, comparison, contrast, emphasis conclusion, summary, additional information, or clarity:

Location	*across, around, away from, beyond, in back of, over, outside*
Time	*while, first, during, next, as soon as, finally, till, at, after*
Comparison	*in the same way, likewise, also, similarly*
Contrast	*although, on the other hand, yet, however*

Emphasis	*to repeat, in fact, for this reason, again*
Summary	*as a result, therefore, in conclusion, to sum up, all in all*
More information	*additionally, besides, for instance, likewise, along with*
Clarity	*in other words, for instance, that is, put another way*

Other ways to unify a paragraph include:

- Repeating words from one sentence to the next:

  The patient was *examined* in the emergency room. On *examination*, the patient's chest and lungs sounded relatively clear.

  The medical history contained many *errors*. An incorrect spelling of the patient's surname was one of the major *errors*.

- Using pronouns that refer back to a noun in a previous sentence:

  The *nurse instructor* insisted that her students use *medical abbreviations* correctly. *She* gave the class a test on *them* daily.

- Repeating a sentence structure:

  A diagnostic report describes the pathological findings of a sample of tissue. The *MRI uses* electromagnetic energy to produce images of body tissue.

- Substituting another word in place of a previous one:

  The *Hb, Hct, WBC,* and *RBC* are normal. The *complete blood count (CBC)* is normal.

- Stating at the beginning of a sentence that there are a particular number of points to be mentioned:

  According to Dr. Elizabeth Kubler-Ross, patients facing death pass through *five* stages. *The first* stage is denial and *the second* is anger.

Medical Spelling

Become familiar with the spelling of the following words:

affect	defuse
Alzheimer's disease	diffuse
arrhythmia	effect
aural	elicit
cite	explicit
coarse	facial
complement	fascial
compliment	illicit
course	implicit
cytology	infarction

infraction	petal
keratosis	profusion
ketosis	reflex
moral	reflux
morale	sight
oral	somatic
osteopenia	vesical
ostalgia	vesicle
pedal	waive
perfusion	wave

Paragraph Study Summary

Types of Paragraphs

Narrative	Relates a story or series of events, usually in chronological order.
Descriptive	Describes details, ideas, actions, settings, or persons.
Expository	Informs, explains, or defines something.
Persuasive	Urges the reader to follow a certain course of action, deal with an issue, or state an opinion about a debatable issue.

Paragraph structure

Topic sentence	Introduces the reader to the main idea.
Supporting sentences	Comprise the details, facts, examples, and questions that support the topic sentence.
Concluding sentence	Brings the paragraph to conclusion.
Paragraph organization	The orderly arrangement of sentences.
Time	Organizes by time.
Logic	Organizes by familiar to unfamiliar, simple to complex, general to specific.
Location	Arranges from left to right, top to bottom, and edge to center.
Deduction	Starts with the general and goes to the specific.
Induction	Starts with specific and goes to the general.
Cause and effect	Connects results of something to an event or fact.
Comparison	Measures one subject against another subject.
Definition	Explains words or ideas in clear fashion.

Paragraph unity	Methods:
The manner in which sentences are formed smoothly, sensibly, and logically.	—Repeat words from one sentence to another. —Use pronouns that refer back to another noun. —Repeat sentence structure. —Substitute new words in place of previous ones. —Use transition words.

Skills Review

1. Write and organize two paragraphs. Here are a few topic suggestions: Why are you studying in the medical profession at this time? What hospital experience do you remember? What was your most memorable experience at the doctor's office?

2. Write a longer piece on your chosen topic, approximately three to five paragraphs.

Identify the correct word:

1. Pertaining to the ears ____________________ (oral, aural)

2. Having to do with the face ____________________ (facial, fascial)

3. Pertaining to the foot ____________________ (petal, pedal)

4. Mental condition with respect to courage, discipline, and willingness to endure hardship ____________________ (moral, morale)

5. To voluntarily postpone, to relinquish ____________________ (wave, waive)

6. The study of cells ____________________ (somatic, cytology)

7. Pertaining to fibrous membranes that cover, support, and separate muscles ____________________ (facial, fascial)

8. Not allowed by law ____________________ (illicit, elicit)

9. To be revealed, to extract, to draw forth ____________________ (elicit, illicit)

10. The passing of a fluid through spaces, supplying tissues or organs with nutrients by injecting blood ____________________ (perfusion, profusion)

11. Pouring forth with a great lavish supply ____________________ (perfusion, profusion)

12. Pertaining to or shaped like a bladder ____________________ (vesible, vesical)

Circle the correctly spelled word in each line:

1. complament	complument	compliment	complment
2. Alxhiemers	Alzheimer's	Alzhimers	Alzhimmers
3. ostealgia	ostalgia	ostialgia	osstalgia
4. arrhythmia	arrithmya	arthythmia	arrythmia
5. karatosis	keratosis	ceratosis	kerotitis
6. rephix	reflux	rephulx	refulx
7. infraxtion	infracshun	infarction	inpharction
8. corse	coarse	korse	coussre
9. fascial	fasial	facsial	fassial
10. purfusion	pirfusion	perfushun	perfusion

Translate medical abbreviations using a medical dictionary or appendix.

1. VD ____________________
2. VDRL ____________________
3. v/o ____________________
4. w/c ____________________
5. WNL ____________________
6. $\bar{p}$ ____________________
7. STAT ____________________
8. PWB ____________________
9. POMR ____________________
10. postop ____________________

Section Three

Writing Skills

Chapter 11

Additional Guidelines for Effective Writing

Objectives

Upon completion of this chapter, the student should be able to:

- implement the five stages of the writing process
- apply the criteria of a good writing style
- understand the advantages and disadvantages of writing on the computer
- spell various medical terms
- translate various medical abbreviations and symbols

The Writing Process

The most important word in the preceding subtitle is the word *process.* A process is a series of steps from beginning to end for achieving a desired result. Writing becomes easier when broken down into manageable steps. A process is not a one-step operation that magically produces a finished product on the first attempt. Many people wrongfully assume that once something is written, it is acceptable and the task is over. Whether a beginner or experienced writer, the implementation of all steps in the writing process is crucial to successful documentation. Dr. Seuss, a prestigious writer of children's literature, pondered hours and days on which preposition (to, of, for, by) conveyed the best meaning and rhythm.

The writing process includes five steps: prewriting, writing, rewriting, finalizing, and proofreading. These steps remain the same for any type of writing: a single sentence, narrative, speech, proposal, instruction, summary, description, paragraph, short story, novel, report, memo, or medical documentation. To demonstrate the steps of the writing process, we use a short paragraph on legal issues in health care as an example.

Step One: Prewriting

The prewriting stage is the planning stage during which an outline of everything the author wants to write about the topic is prepared. At this initial step, the writer thinks about the reading audience and begins to focus more clearly on the subject. Details are jotted down in any order. If necessary, the author researches and limits the amount and

TOPIC	Legal Issues Affecting Health Care
SPECIFICS	Negligence Asault and batery Invasion of pivacy
NOTES	Research definitions Place issues in alphabetical order Have a good opening and closing sentence Keep the language simple Limit paragraph to five or six sentences

Figure 11-1 Prewriting Sample

length of writing. Correct spelling is not necessary at this stage. See Figure 11-1 for a sample of the prewriting process.

Step Two: Writing

In the second step of the writing process, a pencil is placed on paper or fingers on the keyboard. The task is to start writing and keep it flowing. Forget about spelling, grammar, or punctuation at this point. Do not try to make things perfect. Just write. Let anything happen. Present facts or ideas about the topic. See Figure 11-2 for a sample of step two.

> The Patients bill of Rights require that patients be treated with respect Some violations against patients rights are asault, negligence, invasion of privacy, verble abuse. Asault is verble or physical treats that cause harm, injury or fear. Failure to give proper care to patients is called negligense. Discussing information about patients publically without there soncent is unlawful. Failure to obey these areas make one lible or legally responsible.

Figure 11-2 Writing Sample

Step Three: Rewriting

Read the first draft. Does it say what it is meant to say? Is the message clear and complete? Are facts or events in the right order? Does the writing follow the plan established in the prewriting stage? Concentrate on *each* word. Now correct grammar, spelling, and punctuation. (When using a computer, never depend solely on it to check spelling and grammar.) Change what needs to be changed. If necessary, consult others for feedback. Notice any satisfaction or discomfort that comes with reading the words. If there is discomfort, more work is needed. Review Figure 11-3 for the rewriting phase.

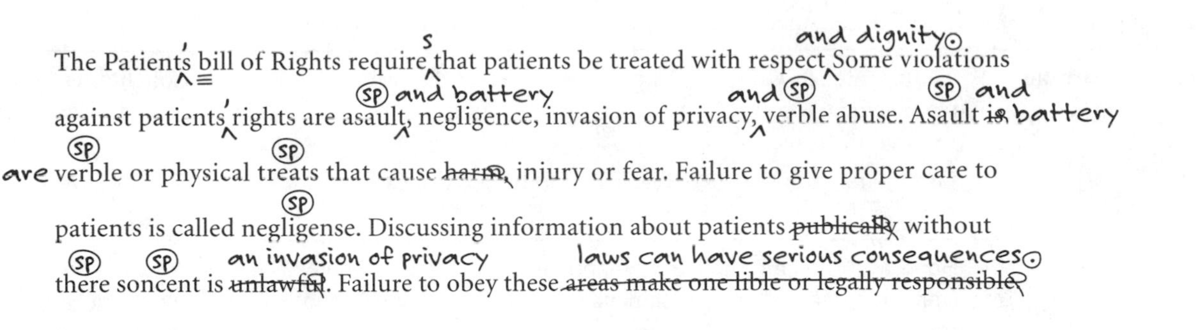
and dignity

The Patients bill of Rights require that patients be treated with respect Some violations

and battery and and

against patients rights are asault, negligence, invasion of privacy, verble abuse. Assault is battery

are verble or physical treats that cause harm, injury or fear. Failure to give proper care to

patients is called negligense. Discussing information about patients publically without

an invasion of privacy laws can have serious consequences

there soncent is unlawful. Failure to obey these areas make one lible or legally responsible

Figure 11-3 Rewriting Sample

Step 4: Finalizing

Once you are satisfied with the corrections, rewrite or type the final version. Figure 11-4 shows the result of finalizing your work.

The Patient's Bill of Rights requires that patients be treated with respect and dignity. Some violations against patient's rights are assault and battery, negligence, invasion of privacy, and verbal abuse. Assault and battery are verbal or physical treats that cause injury or fear. Failure to give proper care to patients is called negligence. Discussing information about patients without their consent is an invasion of privacy. Failure to obey these laws can have serious consequences.

Figure 11-4 Finalizing Sample

Step Five: Proofreading

The purpose of proofreading is to check and correct the final printed product. The proofreading stage is not the time to make major changes. It is the time to check for typing errors or slips of the pen. Mistakes reflect a negative image to the reader about the management of the medical office. Patients may assume or conclude that poor office performance means poor patient care. In the final copy of the sample paragraph resulting from step four (Figure 11-4) find the two errors that still remain. See Appendix F for proofreading marks.

In summary, it should be evident that good writing does not just happen. A writer must follow a systematic approach that calls for planning, organizing, writing, evaluating, and revising. Just as you learn to read by reading, you learn to write by writing. Take what you learned about paragraph development in Chapter 10 and integrate it with the writing process just described (see Figure 11-5). Then practice. Writing improves with practice. Practice is the key to successful writing.

General purpose for writing: Educate medical assistants on ways to prevent and control disease			
Step 1: Prewriting Jot down, organize ideas.	Topic sentence: Go from general topic to a specific topic. Limit paragraph to hand washing.	Supporting Sentences: Facts, details to support the topic sentence. How hand washing is done.	Concluding Sentence: Ties related ideas together. Benefit of washing hands.
Step 2: Writing Write without concern for grammar.	Hand washing can limit the spread of germs.	Before and after contact with a pateint, completely wet and soap hands and wrist. Work into a lather. Get between fingers and under the nails. Rince well, lowering hand downward. Dry with a towel. Turn off the water tap with the paper towel. Apply lotion if desire.	Washing hands is an important way to control disease.
Step 3: Rewriting Correct grammar, spelling, make changes, using proofreaders marks.	Hand washing is an important step in limiting the spread of germs.	Before and after contact with a pateint, completely wet and soap hands and wrist. Work into a lather. Get between fingers and under the nails. Rince well, lowering hand downward. Dry with a towel. Turn off the water tap with the paper towel. Apply lotion if desire.	Handwashing is the most effective way to prevent and control disease.
Step 4: Finalizing Type or write final copy.	Hand washing is one important step that helps limit the spread of germs.	Before and after contact with patients completely wet hands and wrist. Work soap into lather, getting between fingers and under nails. Lower hands with fingernails downward and rinse well. Dry hands carefully with a paper towel. Turn off the water tap with a paper towel to avoid any germs on the faucet. Apply location if desired.	Handwashing is the most effective way to prevent and control disease.
Step 5: Proofreading Read aloud for a final check.	OK	Place a comma after "patients" in the first sentence.	Separate "hand washing."

Figure 11-5 Integration of Paragraph Development with the Writing Process

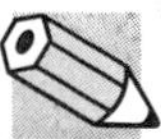

Practice 11-1

Using the five steps of the writing process, write a paragraph of approximately six to eight sentences.

Writing Style

The dictionary defines the word *style* as a manner in which something is said, done, expressed, or performed. Style reveals how a writer thinks and feels about the people and situations that are the subjects of the writing. The two basic rules that apply to all types of writing are:

1. The writing style should be appropriate for the situation.
2. The writing style should be consistent throughout the writing.

Following are some of the criteria of a good writing style:

- *Purpose.* Initially, writers should know their audience and the purpose for which a particular writing task is being done. Is it to persuade, inform, entertain, or explain? Whatever the purpose, it must be clear, original, and focused on the message to be conveyed. What does the writer want the reader to understand? If the writer is not clear about the message, the reader will not be either. Writing is done for someone to read and should immediately engage the reader's interest.

  In a medical office setting, the purpose for writing is to document, transcribe, and organize patients' medical data in order to form a quality environment for good medical care.

> *No matter how technical a subject, all writing is done for human beings by human beings.*
>
> Jacqueline Berke

- *Appropriate Wording.* Writing style is developed from a series of choices that makes the writer's style unique. One of those choices involves the words that are used. Words are combined to convey an intended meaning or attitude. A message with the same meaning can be written in many different ways for different situations:

  His heart is fluttering.

  His heart flutters whenever he sees you.

  His heart is in tachycardia.

  The patient has tachycardia.

  The rate of heart palpitations has reached a serious level.

  This medicine does things to my heart.

  The patient has an increased heart rate.

  My heart is all worked up over this health problem.

  The style of writing for a newspaper is quite different from that of a novel, textbook, romance, research paper, biography, poem, narrative, short story, business letter, autobiography, or medical report. The writing style of the medical profession is unique. In medical documentation, writing is brief and detailed. For example:

  Acetaminophen 2 tabs. q. 4 h.

  Acetaminophen 1000 mg. q. 4 h. p.r.n.

  To be skilled in the style of medical documentation, knowledge of medical terms and abbreviations is of utmost importance. Use words that are precise and concise so the reader can easily understand what is said.

> *Doctors bury their mistakes. Lawyers hang them. Journalists put their mistakes on the front page.*
>
> Anonymous

- *Explicitness.* Good writing avoids generalization and is as specific as possible.

  General Give the patient aspirin for pain.
  Specific Pt. gets ASA 500 mg. q. 4 h. p.r.n. for pain.

General	Patient says he has pain in the back.
Specific	Pt. states he has low back pain in the lumbar region.
General	The patient suffered from pain.
Specific	The patient suffered from a migraine headache.
General	The physician began the treatment.
Specific	The physician reluctantly began the treatment.
General	The patient is not to eat before the exam. Upper GI series is to be done.
Specific	Pt. is n.p.o. after 2 a.m. UGI series in the a.m.
General	The patient is coughing after surgery.
Specific	Pt. is coughing/deep breathing q. 15 min. while awake.

> *Trim sentences, like trim bodies, usually require far more effort than flabby ones.*
>
> Clair Kehrwald Cook

- *Conciseness.* A complete message stated in as few words as possible and without unnecessary words is another feature of good writing style.

Redundant	The pt. was violent, abusive, and was hitting the nurse.
Clearer	Patient showed violent behavior.
Wordy	Place the reports in the file. After the reports are in the file, put them in alphabetical order.
Clearer	File the reports alphabetically.
Wordy	The reason I was late was due to the fact that my alarm clock didn't ring.
Clearer	I was late because I forgot to set the alarm.

> *The beautiful part of writing is that you don't have to get it right the first time, unlike, say, a brain surgeon.*
>
> Robert Cormier

- *Correct Grammar.* The use of good grammar is usually equated with writing well. Although the two are interconnected, one does not necessarily guarantee the other. While it may be useful to learn isolated skills at times, grammatical concepts must be learned by integrating them into the context of writing. Writers must transfer what they learn from studying grammar to their own writing.

- *Smoothness.* The use of transitional words to unite one sentence or paragraph with another helps to eliminate bumps or rough spots. Each sentence or paragraph should lead clearly and logically to the next, providing a smooth flow of ideas.

  The x-rays were negative. *Therefore*, additional testing is unnecessary.

  The patient didn't follow directions when using the medication. *Consequently*, her blood pressure reading was invalid.

- *Inclusive Language.* All types of medical writing should contain gender-free language. At one point in history, nursing was considered only a woman's career and most physicians were men:

  The doctor and his patients . . .   The nurse and her patients . . .

In today's society, the use of nondiscriminating language prevents occupational stereotyping and makes men and women equal.

The hospital employee must sign *his* name.

The hospital employee must sign *her* name.

The hospital employee signed *his/her* name.

Many professionals feel that the *his/her* combination is awkward. Two ways to avoid its use are (1) by changing nouns to their plural form and using the pronoun *their,* and (2) by rewriting the sentence to avoid using a pronoun.

Hospital employees must sign *their* benefit plans.

All hospital employees must sign benefit plans.

Use of gender-free language in written (and spoken) language fosters equality in the workplace. Note how gender-specific terms have changed over the years:

mankind	humankind
chairman	chairperson
housewife	homemaker
my girl/boy	my assistant
policeman	police officer
salesman	salesperson
stewardess	flight attendant

To develop a good writing style requires commitment to the writing process. Writing is hard work and needs constant editing and revising. No matter how experienced a writer, there is always room for improvement. The health-care professional must be committed to the writing process in order to give the task the proper attention it needs and the practice it requires. Practice is the key to becoming a good writer. Practice is what makes good writing better. All writings possess the challenge to improve. Good writing is achieved by working and reworking ideas again and again.

Finally, learning to write well goes beyond good grammar skills, proofreading, revising, and organizing. Developing writing skills also comes from reading the works of good writers.

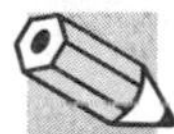

Practice 11-2

Rewrite to simplify these sentences:

1. I can't tell you, Doctor, how I really, really appreciate what you did for me.

   ____

2. Working in the operating room, the nurse did not see the doctor.

   ____

3. Cathy was Dr. Villmare's medical assistant. She work two years for him.

   ____

4. Read the medical report literally, word for word. ____________________

5. It is the hospital's intention to issue bonuses based on a worker's performance.

   ____

6. People who get into accidents on the job are just plain careless. ________________

7. The meeting began at noon and started with a dozen people in attendance.
____

8. May I refer you back to the agreement we made six months ago? ________________

9. As luck would have it, we were fortunate to make a profit. ________________

10. The doctor's handwriting was illegible and difficult to read. ________________

Computer Writing

A computer is a writer's best friend, providing that the writer has keyboard, writing, and computer skills. If competent in two areas, the other one can be learned. Otherwise, using the computer to improve writing may be counterproductive.

The advantages to using a computer far outweigh the disadvantages for many reasons:

- The computer is faster than longhand writing.
- The writer can focus more freely on ideas.
- The writer can endure longer periods of writing time and cover a topic more thoroughly.
- Revisions are easier to make.
- Small and large sections can be added, moved, or deleted.
- Pages have uniform margins and formats.
- Nice touches can be added to work: type styles, italics, bold print, illustrations, tables and charts, and colors.
- Spell check and grammar check help spot errors quickly.
- Printouts are clean and easier to read.

Among the disadvantages are:

- The writer has to continually stop and read what was written.
- Some errors, such as missing words, commas, and periods, are hard to see on the screen.
- For some writers, revising, rereading, and evaluating from the screen is more difficult than from a paper.

Medical Spelling

Become familiar with the spelling of the following words:

absorbent
accessible
accommodation
analysis
analyze
beneficial
canceled
conscious
comparative
convalescent
deficiency
diarrhea

eligible	prescription
flatulence	procedure
hemorrhage	quantity
hygiene	recurrence
inadvertently	referral
infectious	reiterated
intermittent	rheumatism
irritated	severity
irrigated	successful
judgment	sufficient
necessary	susceptible
occurrence	suture
opportunity	tachycardia
palliative	technique
perseverance	umbilicus
precede	xiphoid

Additional Guidelines for Effective Writing Study Summary

The Writing Process:	a series of steps for achieving effective writing.
1. Prewriting	Outline the topics to include in the writing.
2. Writing	Write and keep it flowing, without regard to correct spelling, grammar, or punctuation.
3. Rewriting	Correct errors and determine if the message is clear.
4. Finalizing	Write or type the final copy.
5. Proofreading	Check the final version for remaining errors.
Writing Style:	the manner in which something is expressed.
Characteristics of Good Writing	
Purpose	Understand why a message is written.
Appropriate wording	Use the style that fits the message.
Explicitness	Avoid generalizations and be specific.
Conciseness	State the message once and in as few words as possible.
Correct grammar	Transfer grammar skills to writing.
Smoothness	Use transitional words to unite sentences.
Inclusive language	Use gender-free language.

Skills Review

1. List the five steps of the writing process in their correct order.

2. Describe the work of each step in the writing process.

3. Using these five steps, write three or four original paragraphs that incorporate some of the characteristics of a good writing style.

____

____

____

____

____

____

4. List four advantages and two disadvantages of using the computer to write.

____

____

____

____

____

____

Answer true or false to the following statements:

1. A writer with good grammar skills will automatically write well. _____
2. Reading the works of famous authors can help improve one's writing. _____
3. Ordinarily, the works of good experienced writers don't need much revision. _____
4. The purpose of a topic sentence is to tie ideas together. _____
5. For an experienced writer, skipping a stage of the writing process is allowed. _____
6. Writing for health-care personnel consists mainly of transcribing medical manuscripts. _____
7. Correct spelling and grammar are necessary through all phases of the writing process. _____
8. If one word conveys a clear message, use it. _____
9. A broad vocabulary makes reading more interesting. _____

10. The informal writing style for medical personnel should exclude abbreviations. _____

11. Writing should be reworked again and again. _____

12. A writer does not have to proofread if the spell check and grammar check on the computer is used. _____

13. In the first step of the writing process, concern for correct grammar is necessary. _____

14. In medical writing, repeat ideas often to convey the message. _____

15. A series of steps from beginning to end is called a process. _____

16. The writing style for medical documentation is brief and as detailed as possible. _____

Select the best-constructed sentence in each group:

1. A. Because patients pay the bill, invoices are their responsibility.

   B. Invoices are the patients' responsibility

   C. Medical assistants send invoices to patients.

2. A. When the patient was young, the patient had frequent urinary tract infections as a child.

   B. The patient had urinary tract infections as a child.

   C. The patient had frequent urinary tract infections as a child.

3. A. Most likely, the syndrome is viral hepatitis.

   B. I thought the syndrome was viral hepatitis.

   C. The syndrome is thought by me to be most likely viral hepatitis.

4. A. I am thrilled that you referred this pleasant, beautiful patient to me.

   B. Thank you for referring this patient for neurological evaluation.

   C. Thank you for the reference.

5. A. Avoidance of the infection is the best approach.

   B. Avoidance of the infection includes polio vaccination.

   C. Avoidance includes vaccination of anyone with the disease.

Circle the correctly spelled word in each line:

1. perservirance perseverance preseverance preseverance
2. paliative palliative paleative palleative
3. necsesary nessessary necessary necissary
4. prescription perscripition perscription prescishun
5. rhumatism ruematism rhuematism rheumatism
6. acomodation accomodation accommodation acommodation
7. benificial beneficial benefecial beneficle
8. ocurrence occurence occurrance occurrence
9. intermittent interrmittant intermittant intermitant
10. diarhea diarea diarrhhea diarrhea

Translate medical abbreviations using a medical dictionary or appendix.

1. / ____________________
2. FH ____________________
3. $\bar{c}$ ____________________
4. $\bar{s}$ ____________________
5. $>$ ____________________
6. $<$ ____________________
7. $\therefore$ ____________________
8. Δ ____________________
9. Ⓡ ____________________
10. Ⓛ ____________________

Section Four

Applications

Chapter 12

Medical Office Correspondence

Objectives

Upon completion of this chapter, the student should be able to:

- distinguish among the various types of correspondence in the medical office
- implement a simple format when using each type of correspondence
- prepare block and modified block letters with accompanying envelope
- understand the purpose of the memo, e-mail, fax, and phone message
- write and maintain minutes of a business meeting
- write an original letter, memo, phone message, e-mail, and fax
- spell various medical terms
- translate various medical abbreviations and symbols

Writing in the medical office is a highly structured form of communication. Correspondence is a process of sharing medical-related information through standardized letters, memos, reports, and electronic messages. Through these means, both the receiver and the sender have a document that holds more legality than the spoken word. This chapter outlines some of the varied communication tasks that medical professionals need to perform.

The Medical Letter

At one time or another, all medical personnel need to write a medical letter. Written communication requires a basic knowledge of sentence structure, spelling, punctuation, medical terms, and abbreviations, all of which are covered in previous chapters. A medical letter, like other types of writing, requires that the steps of the writing process be implemented. The overall appearance of a medical letter is also important. It should make a favorable impression at first glance. Correspondence is another outward sign reflecting the professionalism of the medical office.

Letter Components

A letter has six basic parts: the heading, inside address, salutation, body, closing, and signature.

Heading

The heading includes the letterhead and the date line. The letterhead is usually commercially printed with a logo, physician's name or medical group, and address. Some may include a telephone number or medical specialty. When using letterhead paper, only the date needs to be typed, including the month, day, and year with no abbreviations. The date is placed *three lines* below the letterhead, flush with the left margin. If there is no letterhead on the paper, the information is typed by the writer. Figure 12-1 shows a sample heading.

VILLES MEDICAL CENTER
One Morey Place
Anywhere, MA 01102
(555) 555-4727 Phone
(555) 555-4000 Fax

July 15, 20XX

Figure 12-1 Heading

Inside Address

The inside address gives the name and address of the person or facility to which the letter is going. It is the mailing address. It is placed *four lines* below the date line, flush with the left margin (Figure 12-2).

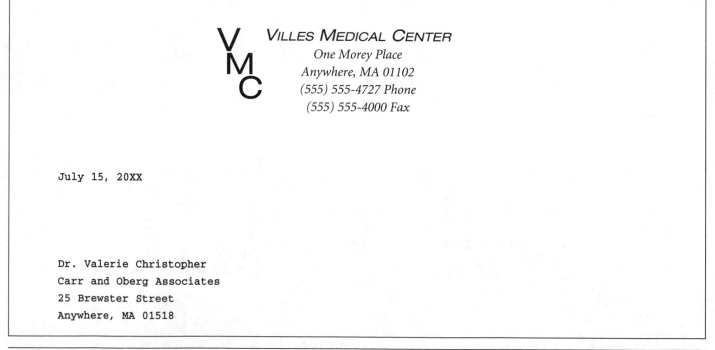

VILLES MEDICAL CENTER
One Morey Place
Anywhere, MA 01102
(555) 555-4727 Phone
(555) 555-4000 Fax

July 15, 20XX

Dr. Valerie Christopher
Carr and Oberg Associates
25 Brewster Street
Anywhere, MA 01518

Figure 12-2 Inside Address

If the title of the person is included in the inside address, it goes after the name on the same line. If the title is too long, place it on the second line.

Examples

Dr. Valerie Christopher, President Carr and Oberg Associates 25 Brewster Street Anywhere, MA 01518	Mary Louise Norman, M.D. Chairperson, Board of Directors 25 Brewster Street Anywhere, MA 01518

Salutation

The salutation is the greeting of the letter. It is placed *two lines* below the inside address, flush with the left margin. A colon (:) follows the salutation (Figure 12-3). All words in the salutation begin with capital letters.

Examples

Firm or Group	Dear Customer Service Representative, Colleagues, Friends, Members of the Search Committee, Gentlemen, Ladies, Editors, Physicians, Students
Special Unknown Person	Dear Personnel Director, Sir, Madame, Clerk of Deeds, Nurse Supervisor
Special Known Persons	Dear Dr. Norman, Nurse Rose, Mr. Oberg, Mary, Miss Leclaire

VMC **VILLES MEDICAL CENTER**
One Morey Place
Anywhere, MA 01102
(555) 555-4727 Phone
(555) 555-4000 Fax

July 15, 20XX

Dr. Valerie Christopher
Carr and Oberg Associates
25 Brewster Street
Anywhere, MA 01518

Dear Dr. Christopher:

Figure 12-3 Salutation

Body

The body of the letter contains the message. The first line of the body is placed *two lines* below the salutation, flush with the left margin (Figure 12-4). The body may have more than one paragraph with double spacing between each paragraph.

VMC

VILLES MEDICAL CENTER
One Morey Place
Anywhere, MA 01102
(555) 555-4727 Phone
(555) 555-4000 Fax

July 15, 20XX

Dr. Valerie Christopher
Carr and Oberg Associates
25 Brewster Street
Anywhere, MA 01518

Dear Dr. Christopher:

Thank you for referring your patient, Mr. Burt Weaver, to Villes Medical Center. Mr. Weaver's psychological status on his initial evaluation necessitated a semiemergency evaluation. I diagnosed the patient as having an adjustment disorder and major depression. He was placed on antidepressant medication for three months.

During this time, Mr. Weaver also participated in six group sessions and ten individual psychotherapy sessions before reaching his maximum rehabilitation. At the time of his discharge, Mr. Weaver was made aware that he could return to Villes Medical Center at any time, if warranted.

If you have any further questions, please call my office at (555) 555-4727.

Figure 12-4 Body

Sometimes in medical correspondence, a subject line is used to call attention to what's important in the letter. The subject line is typed two lines before the salutation, flush with the left margin in the block style (Figure 12-5). The subject line in most cases is a patient's name or medical topic and is considered part of the body of a letter.

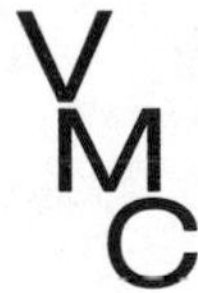

VILLES MEDICAL CENTER
One Morey Place
Anywhere, MA 01102
(555) 555-4727 Phone
(555) 555-4000 Fax

July 15, 20XX

Dr. Valerie Christopher
Carr and Oberg Associates
25 Brewster Street
Anywhere, MA 01518

Mr Burt Weaver

Dear Dr. Christopher:

Thank you for referring. . . .

Figure 12-5 Use of Subject Line

Closing and Signature

The closing is the leave-taking part of the letter. It is typed on the *second line* below the last line of the body. Only the first word in the closing is capitalized. A comma is placed after the last word.

Examples

Yours truly,	Sincerely,	Thank you,
Very truly yours,	Sincerely yours,	With best wishes,
With best regards,	Cordially,	Respectfully yours,

The signature is handwritten in ink right after and *directly below* the closing. In addition, the writer's name is typed *four lines* directly below the closing (Figure 12-6). The typed name may also include the writer's position.

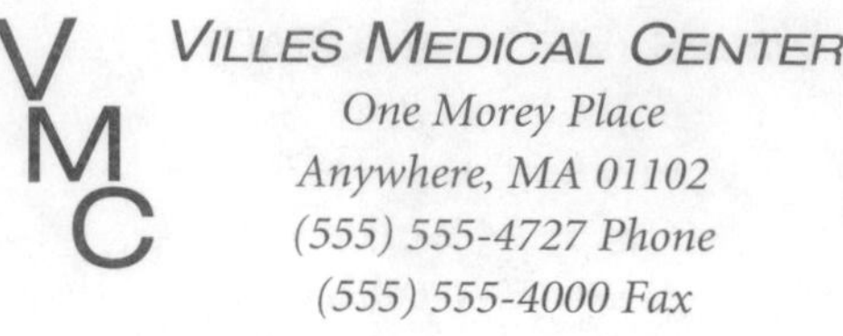

July 15, 20XX

Dr. Valerie Christopher
Carr and Oberg Associates
25 Brewster Street
Anywhere, MA 01518

Dear Dr. Christopher:

Thank you for referring your patient, Mr. Burt Weaver, to Villes Medical Center. Mr. Weaver's psychological status on his initial evaluation necessitated a semiemergency evaluation. I diagnosed the patient as having an adjustment disorder and major depression. He was placed on antidepressant medication for three months.

During this time, Mr. Weaver also participated in six group sessions and ten individual psychotherapy sessions before reaching his maximum rehabilitation. At the time of his discharge, Mr. Weaver was made aware that he could return to Villes Medical Center at any time, if warranted.

If you have any further questions, please call my office at (555) 555-4727.

Yours truly,

Dr. Mary Louise Norman

Figure 12-6 Closing and Signature

Other Notations

If the author of the letter did not type it, the typist's initials are typed on the second line below the typewritten signature, flush with the left margin. If there are enclosures with the letter, an "Enc." is typed directly below the typist's initials. If copies of a letter are given to other people, "CC:" and the name of the person to whom the copy is sent should be typed on a new line following "Enc.," or the typist's initials if there is no "Enc."

Example

Yours truly,

Dr. Mary Louise Norman

LNV
Enc.
CC: Mary Pat Leonard, MD

If the office's name and address does not appear at the top of the stationery, type this information under the writer's typed name (or title) following the signature.

Example

Dr. Mary Louis Norman
Villes Medical Center
One Morey Place
Anywhere, MA 01102
(555) 555-4727
(555) 555-4000 Fax

If a letter runs longer than one page, the heading on the second page should contain the name of the writer, the page number, and the date. It should begin flush with the left margin and can be typed across or stacked.

Examples

(1) Mary Louise Norman, M.D. -2- July 15, 20XX

(2) Mary Louise Norman, M.D.
Page 2
July 15, 20XX

(3) Mary Louise Norman, M.D.
Page 2
July 15, 20XX
Subject: Mr. Burt Weaver

Formats and Presentation of Letters

The two most common styles of formal letters are the block style and the modified block style. The difference between the two is that the block style has no indentations and the modified block does. The date, closing, and signature are indented to the middle of the page. The example letter used in this chapter to explain the basic letter parts is the block style (Figure 12-7). A modified block example of the same letter is also included (Figure 12-8).

Most medical offices and clinics use official letterhead paper. The standard size is 8½-by-11-inch or 5½-by-8½-inch paper for shorter notes. Whether using letterhead stationery or plain stationery, the margins must be equal on the top, bottom, and left and right sides, usually one inch. Margins can be compared to the matting on a picture. Margins are the frame of the letter. Letters are typed single spaced unless the message is extremely short, in which case double spacing is acceptable.

To be most effective, the letter should be as short as possible. A single page is preferable.

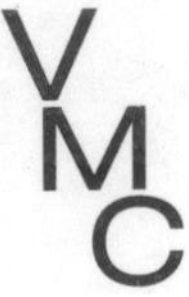

VILLES MEDICAL CENTER
One Morey Place
Anywhere, MA 01102
(555) 555-4727 Phone
(555) 555-4000 Fax

July 15, 20XX

Dr. Valerie Christopher
Carr and Oberg Associates
25 Brewster Street
Anywhere, MA 01518

Dear Dr. Christopher:

Thank you for referring your patient, Mr. Burt Weaver, to Villes Medical Center. Mr. Weaver's psychological status on his initial evaluation necessitated a semiemergency evaluation. I diagnosed the patient as having an adjustment disorder and major depression. He was placed on antidepressant medication for three months.

During this time, Mr. Weaver also participated in six group sessions and ten individual psychotherapy sessions before reaching his maximum rehabilitation. At the time of his discharge, Mr. Weaver was made aware that he could return to Villes Medical Center at any time, if warranted.

If you have any further questions, please call my office at (555) 555-4727.

Yours truly,

Dr. Mary Louise Norman

LNV

Figure 12-7 Block Style letter

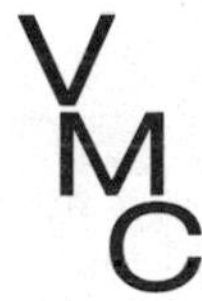

VILLES MEDICAL CENTER
One Morey Place
Anywhere, MA 01102
(555) 555-4727 Phone
(555) 555-4000 Fax

July 15, 20XX

Dr. Valerie Christopher
Carr and Oberg Associates
25 Brewster Street
Anywhere, MA 01518

Dear Dr. Christopher:

Thank you for referring your patient, Mr. Burt Weaver, to Villes Medical Center. Mr. Weaver's psychological status on his initial evaluation necessitated a semiemergency evaluation. I diagnosed the patient as having an adjustment disorder and major depression. He was placed on antidepressant medication for three months.

During this time, Mr. Weaver also participated in six group sessions and ten individual psychotherapy sessions before reaching his maximum rehabilitation. At the time of his discharge, Mr. Weaver was made aware that he could return to Villes Medical Center at any time, if warranted.

If you have any further questions, please call my office at (555) 555-4727.

Yours truly,

Dr. Mary Louise Norman

LNV

Figure 12-8 Modified Block Letter

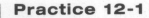

Practice 12-1

Match the terms with their definitions:

1. body _______
2. written signature _______
3. heading _______
4. closing _______
5. inside address _______
6. letterhead stationery _______
7. typed signature _______
8. block style letter _______
9. salutation _______
10. modified block letter _______

A. leave-taking of the letter
B. typed name of sender
C. the greeting
D. parts of the letter are indented
E. everything in letter begins at the left margin
F. company's name and address printed on stationery
G. message of the letter
H. person and address to whom the letter is written
I. address of person writing the letter
J. written in ink after the closing

Folding the Letter

The manner in which the letter is folded depends on the size of the envelope used. The following folds apply to an 8½-by-11-inch letter.

Business Envelope (9½ by 4³⁄₁₆ inches)

Step One Bring the bottom third of the paper up and fold.

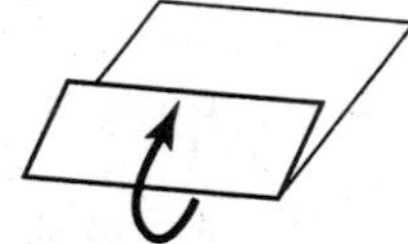

Step Two Fold the top third to within about ⅜ inch of fold made in step one.

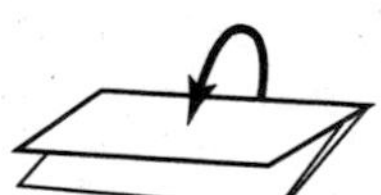

Step Three Insert the folded edge of the letter into the envelope.

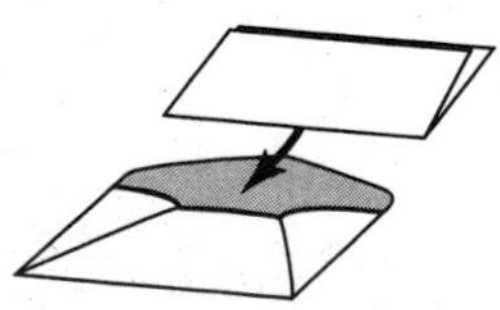

Use the Envelope to Get the Folds Right

Step One Slip the top edge of the letter all the way up under the flap.

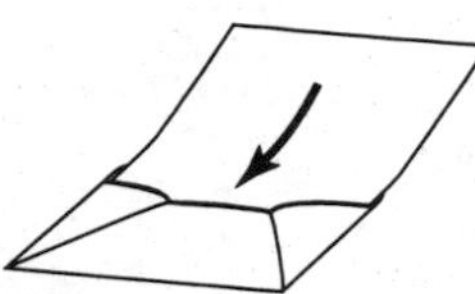

Step Two Fold the bottom part of the letter so that the bottom edge of the letter and the envelope align.

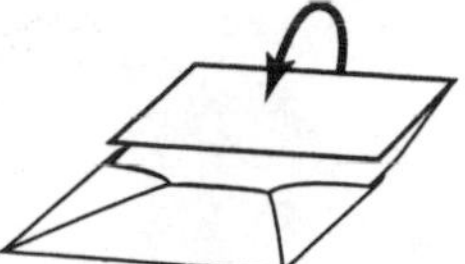

Step Three Pull the letter out from under the flap of the envelope and fold the top over to within 3/8 inch of the bottom fold.

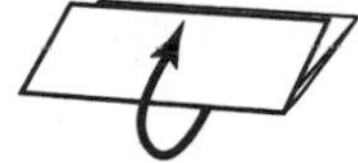

Smaller Envelopes

Step One Fold from the bottom to a quarter of an inch from the top.

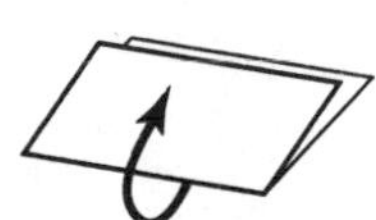

Step Two Fold over the right-hand third of the letter.

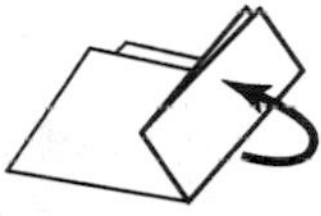

Step Three The left side is folded over that fold.

Step Four Insert the letter with the fold at the bottom of the envelope.

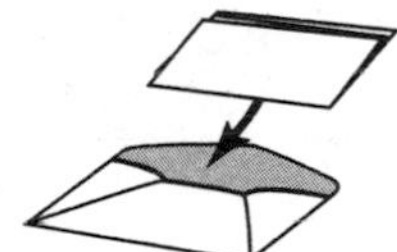

Envelopes with Windows

Step One Bring the bottom third of the letter up and fold.

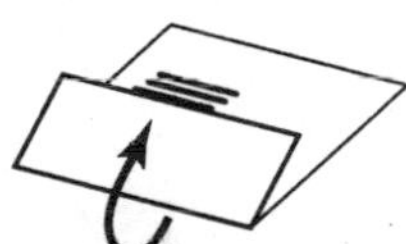

Step Two Fold the top part *back* to the fold made in step one.

Step Three Insert the letter toward the *front* of the envelope so that the mailing address shows through the window.

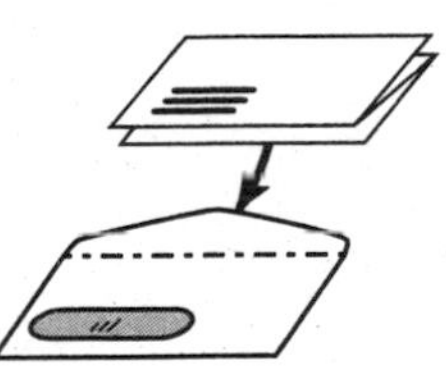

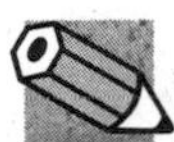

Practice 12-2

Number these folds in the correct order.

A.

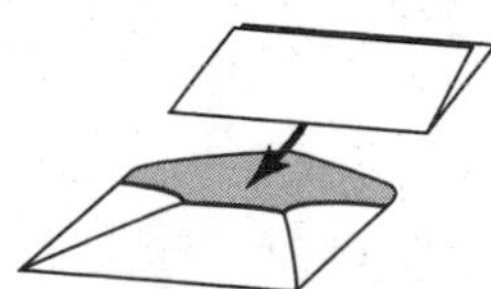

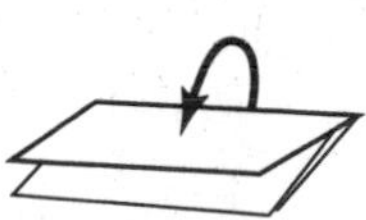

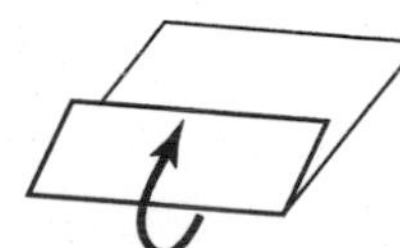

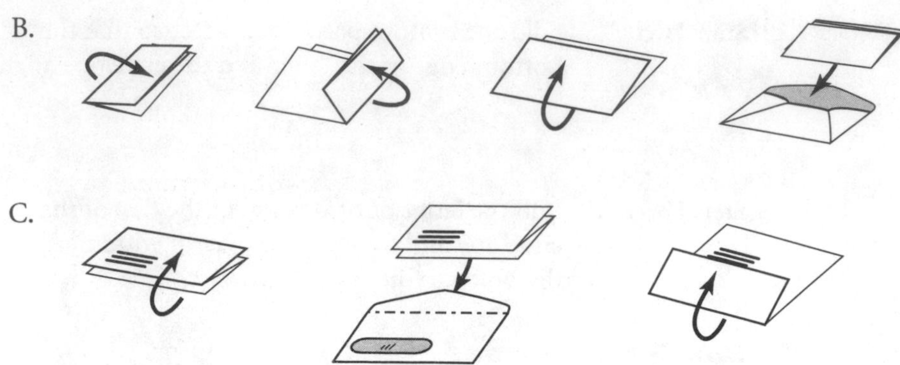

Addressing the Envelope

For envelopes with a preprinted return address, only the recipient's address is typed. This address should correspond to the inside address on the letter. Begin the address in the middle of the envelope, slightly to the right. Use proper titles, including the first name or initial or the person to whom the letter is sent. Directly below that line is the street address. The third line contains the city, state, and zip code. If the envelope has no return address, it must be typed in the upper left corner. See Figure 12-9 for a properly typed envelope.

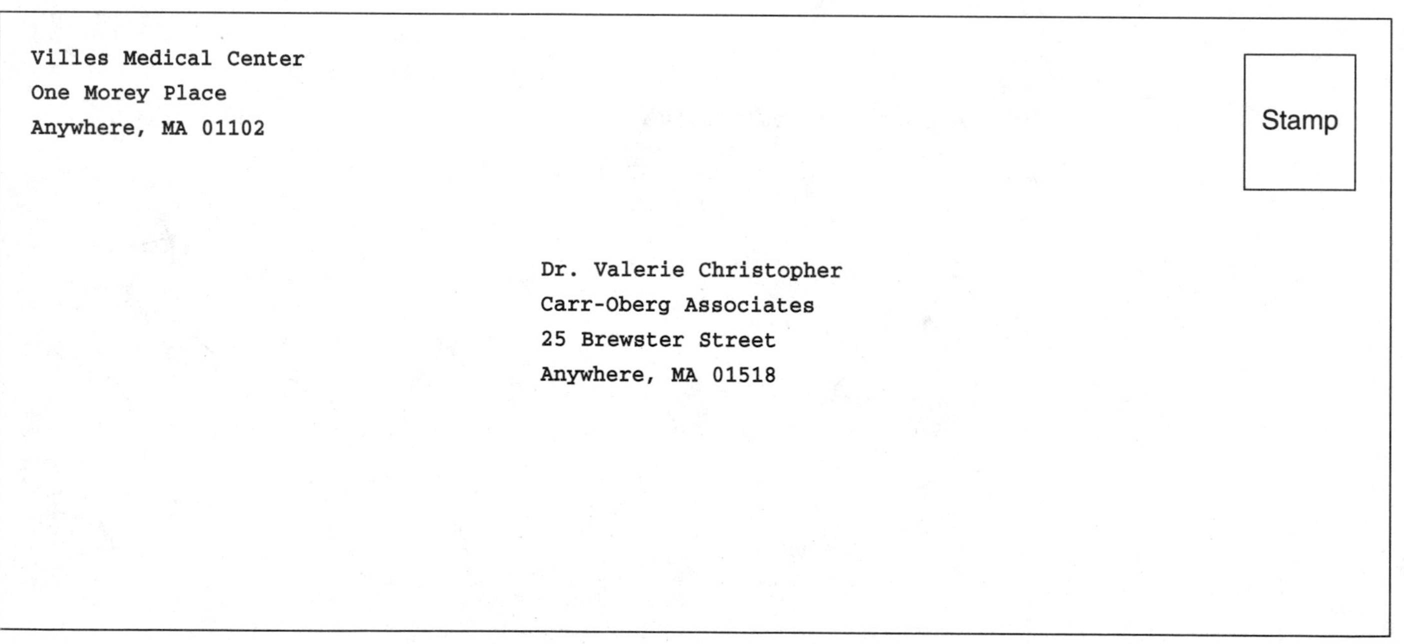

Villes Medical Center
One Morey Place
Anywhere, MA 01102
Stamp
Dr. Valerie Christopher
Carr-Oberg Associates
25 Brewster Street
Anywhere, MA 01518

Figure 12-9 Addressing an Envelope

The Interoffice Memorandum

The interoffice memo is a written message sent to coworkers *in the same company or organization.* Its purpose is to expedite the flow of all types of information; ask or answer questions; describe procedures or policies; remind people of meetings or appointments; or list names, schedules, written records, pronouncements, or work activities.

Although memos are most often used for short communication, their length can vary from one sentence to many pages. Because they are intended for internal circulation, they are less formal than a business letter and do not include the inside address, salutation, or complimen tary close.

Structure of a Memo

Some organizations have special printed forms for interoffice memos, but a plain piece of paper is sufficient. The format for the content of a memo must be very simple. Consider this structure as an example:

To:	(the person to whom the message is written)
From:	(the name of the person writing the message)
Subject: (or **Re:**)	(the precise purpose or topic of the memo)
Date:	(month, day, and year the memo is written)

(The message of the memo follows.)

In large facilities, another category may be added after the "From" line; namely, "Dept./Floor/Ext."

Writing the Memo

The writing style of a memo is direct, concise, and clear. The language is plain and simple, with short sentences averaging about 15 words. The memo must be written so readers understand the message. It is sent only to those for whom the message applies. It should look attractive, command attention, and entice the reader.

The most important message of the memo is stated in the first line, followed by any necessary detailed or supportive information. In addition to narrative paragraphs, facts may be listed with numbers or bullets. Make directives and requests specific. Avoid vague messages like, "get back to me about this matter." Replace it with, "call me Tuesday morning, July 30."

The name or initials of the writer appear after "From" in the heading of the memo, yet some people prefer to sign their name below the final line of the body. If added, the signature is always more effective when it is handwritten.

Before closing the body of the memo, state any task or positive result that the writer might expect from the reader. At the end of the message, a "CC:" or "ENC:" may be added, if applicable. See Figure 12-10 for an example of a properly written memo.

VMC VILLES MEDICAL CENTER
INTEROFFICE MEMO

Date: August 1, 20xx

To: Office Medical Assistants

From: Rose Villes, R.N., Office Manager

Subject: Upgrade of Computer Systems

Computer World is giving a training workshop on the MedSoft Computer Program that BMC plans to implement before September 15. Here are the details:

Tuesday, July 15, from 9:00 a.m .to 4:00 p.m.

Second Floor Conference Room

Read the enclosed brochure about the program before attending the workshop.

CC: Dr. Luke Christopher

Enc.

Figure 12-10 Sample Memo

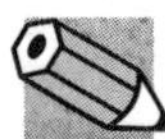

Practice 12-3

Write an interoffice memo that includes this information:

- change in office hours from 8 a.m. to 5 p.m. to 9 a.m. to 4 p.m.
- new hours effective only during the week between Christmas and New Year's
- applies to all staff members
- the message is from Dr. Sarah to staff members

VMC VILLES MEDICAL CENTER

INTEROFFICE MEMO

Date:

To:

From:

Subject:

Electronic Mail

Electronic mail, or e-mail, is a computer-to-computer communication system that transmits messages from one point to another anywhere in the world. This medium is popular because it is convenient, fast and less expensive than a phone call. e-mail can also include any type of text, files, or other documents as part of the message.

E-Mail Guidelines

1. Write only the main message.
2. Put the most important information first.
3. Make the message short, complete, and accurate.
4. Write an attention-getting opening sentence.

5. Limit the message to one screen.
6. Use correct grammar.
7. Proofread the message before sending it. Professionalism is important in e-mail.
8. Save a copy if a record is needed.
9. Eliminate unnecessary closing.
10. Just as e-mail can be sent, e-mail can also be received. Check the office e-mail two or three times a day and respond to incoming messages promptly.

Figure 12-11 gives an example of a properly prepared e-mail.

To:	Lorry Villes, R.N.
From:	Mary Louise Norman, M.D.
Subject:	Staff Meeting, March 5, 20XX, 9 a.m.
CC:	Louis Villes, Chairperson
Date:	February 17, 20XX

Add three additional topics to the agenda for the March 5 meeting. The topics are:

1. Written policies regarding safety procedures
2. Documentation procedures update
3. New computer software needs

If you have any questions, call me at ext. 229.

Figure 12-11 E-mail Format

Facsimile

Written communication often includes more than letters and memos. A facsimile, or fax, machine is an electronic device that transmits documents, drawings, and photographs as *exact* reproductions. The fax is standard equipment in the medical office today and is an excellent way to disseminate valuable medical information among medical facilities and professionals.

In formal professional situations, a cover sheet should accompany any electronically transmitted message or document. Medical offices usually have their own cover sheet format with all necessary information, as follows:

- The name, phone number, and fax number (or extension if applicable) of the sender
- The name, title, department, company, and fax number of the recipient
- The date the fax is sent and the number of pages
- Any written instructions, message, or other information

Figure 12-12 is an example of a fax cover sheet.

One Morey Place
Anywhere, MA 01102
(555) 555-4727 Phone
(555) 555-444 FAX

VMC VILLES MEDICAL CENTER

FAX Cover Sheet

To: Carol LeClaire From: VMC
FAX: 555-555-4444 Date: 6-30-20XX
Phone: 555-4279 Pages: 7
(Including cover sheet.)

Comments

The pathology report you requested on Carlos Rodriguez is enclosed.

Figure 12-12 Sample Fax Cover Sheet

Phone Messages

Most medical offices have an interoffice phone message form that staff members complete when someone cannot be reached by phone. The form is designed to contain all the necessary information without having to write too much. Pertinent information consists of the caller's name and phone number; the name of the person called; the date, time, and purpose of the call; a short message, and the name of the person who took the message. Figure 12-13 is an example of a phone message form.

To Dr. Valerie Christopher
Date 2-18-00 Time 9 am

WHILE YOU WERE OUT
PHONE MESSAGE

M Mark Villes, M.D.
Of Villes Medical Center
Phone 555-5551 Ext 222

	Telephoned		Called to see you.
✓	Please call back.		Returned your call.
	Will call again.		Urgent

MESSAGE
Called regarding a
meeting on
March 31 at 5 p.m.

Beverly Berc, CMA

Figure 12-13 Sample Phone Message

The important thing to remember about phone messages is to deliver them promptly. The efficiency and professionalism of the medical office requires that persons receive information in a timely manner. Be sure the handwritten message is legible.

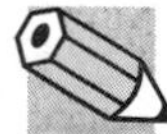

Practice 12-4

Indicate by letter (A–F) the choices of communication under the circumstances described.

A. in person
B. by telephone
C. by fax machine
D. by memo
E. by e-mail
F. by letter

1. ________ Send a report to the hospital as soon as possible.
2. ________ Need an immediate answer for a person in another hospital across town.
3. ________ Laboratory results reported to the physician.
4. ________ A short update is sent to the primary physician about a referred patient.

5. ________ The time and date for a meeting with four different hospital finance directors was changed.

6. ________ A nurse has to cancel and reschedule the doctor's afternoon appointments.

7. ________ Send a message to three other people in the same facility.

8. ________ A CMA is interviewed for a job.

9. ________ The doctor needs a copy of the CMA's resume.

10. ________ Send a brief message across the city.

Minutes of a Meeting

Medical personnel may be expected to type the minutes of a meeting. Minutes are an official (and sometimes legal) summary record of events and decisions that occur during the meeting. Asking *who, what, where, when,* and *why* about the meeting simplifies the process. All questions need not be answered. These questions are only a tool for getting at the important information. Record only what was done at a meeting and not what was said.

Who	Who attends the meeting? Who is absent? Who is responsible for carrying out tasks? Who chairs the meeting? Who is secretary? Who distributes the minutes? Who reminds people of the next meeting?
What	What happens at the meeting? What decisions were made? What was the meeting about? What is the agenda of this meeting or the next meeting?
Where	Where is the meeting? Where is the next meeting?
When	When is the meeting? When is the follow-up meeting? When does this decision take effect?
Why	Why did the group make the decision? Why were some people absent?

Like other forms of written communication, a structured model of writing minutes is necessary to ensure a consistent style. Minutes are usually summarized in three components: a heading, a body, and a conclusion (Figure 12-14).

VMC

```
Villes Medical Center
Office Staff Meeting
Conference Room
October 11, 20XX
2-4 p.m.

Chairperson–Rose Villes, R.N., Office Manager
Secretary–Norbert Oberg, R.N.

1.

2.

3.

Next Meeting–        December 17, 20XX
                     2-4 p.m.
                     Conference Room
```

Figure 12-14 Minutes of a Meeting

Heading	Name of organization
	Purpose of meeting
	Date, time, and place of meeting
	Chairperson and secretary
	Names of those present and absent
	Approval of previous meeting's minutes
Body	Paragraph(s) on subject matters regarding decisions, rulings, events, data
Conclusion	Time and place of next meeting
	Agenda
	Chairperson and secretary

Medical Spelling

Become familiar with the spelling of the following words:

asymmetrical	committee
catastrophic	compliance

conscientious
credentials
diuresis
evidence
forensic
granulocyte
guidelines
hemoptysis
implement
incidence
incidentally
indispensable
infusion
intervention
jaundice
itinerary
kinesiology
legality
metastasis
observation
parameters
periodicals
peripheral
personal
personnel
phlegm
protocol
quandary
recommendations
recuperation
repression
schedule
standardize
thyroid
tourniquet
vaccination
varicose veins
viscosity
xanthosis

Medical Office Correspondence Study Summary

Medical Letter Format

Heading

VMC
VILLES MEDICAL CENTER
One Morey Place
Anywhere, MA 01102
(555) 555-4727 Phone
(555) 555-4000 Fax

(3 spaces)

June 5, 20XX — Date

(4 spaces)

Mary LeClair
Anystreet
Anywhere, MA 00000

Name and address of the person receiving the mail

(2 spaces)

	Dear Mrs. LeClair	Salutation
(2 spaces)		
	The purpose of this letter .... end of letter.	Body—Message of the letter
(2 spaces)		
	Sincerely,	Closing—Leaving-taking
(4 spaces)		Written signature
	Valerie Christopher, M.D.	Typed signature—author of the letter
(2 spaces)		
	VC: lnv	Typists Initials
(2 spaces)		
	cc: Dr. Michael Paul	cc—Others receiving copy
(2 spaces)		
	Enc. Consultation report	Enc.—Enclosures (notations follow in this order)

Other Written Communication

Type of Communication	Definition	Format/Structure
Memo	A written message to coworkers in the same company	**To:** **From:** **Re:** **Date:**
E-mail	A computer-to-computer communication system that transmits messages electronically	To: From: Subject: CC: (optional) Date:
Fax	An electronic device that transmits documents, drawings, and photos as exact reproductions	Cover sheet with name, phone number and fax number of sender; name, title, company, and fax number of recipient; date and number of pages; any message
Phone message	A message from a caller to someone not present to receive the call	Name of person called; caller's name and phone number; date, time, purpose of call; message, name of person who took the message

Type of Communication	Definition	Format/Structure
Minutes of a meeting	A summary of events and decisions that occur at meetings:	
	Heading	Name of organization Purpose of meeting Date, time, and place, of meeting Chairperson and secretary Names of those present and absent Approval of previous meeting's minutes
	Body	Paragraph(s) on subject matters regarding decisions, rulings, events, data
	Conclusion	Time and place of next meeting Agenda Chairperson and secretary

Skills Review

Indicate whether these statements are true or false:

1. The most important procedure in any type of written communication is to follow all steps in the writing process. __________
2. The size stationery used for most medical letters is 11 by 15 inches. __________
3. A full heading is not necessary on medical letterhead paper. __________
4. The modified block style of a letter has no indentations. __________
5. "Yours truly" is a common salutation in a medical letter. __________
6. "CC:" in a letter means a copy was sent to additional persons. __________
7. The number of folds for an 8½-by-11-inch paper is three. __________
8. An inside address is omitted in a memo. __________
9. Another word for memo is memorandum. __________
10. "Re:" and "Subject:" have the same meaning. __________
11. To send an e-mail is more expensive than using the telephone. __________
12. A cover letter is not necessary when sending a fax. __________
13. Phone messages may be written in longhand. __________

14. Write down everything that happens when taking minutes for a meeting. ________

15. The full block letter does not have indentations ________

Write the correct word from the list on the line after the phrase that defines it.

letter	memo	fax	table of contents	e-mail
minutes	telephone	envelope	full block letter	modified block letter

1. Electronic device that sends exact reproductions ________________

2. A formal account in detail ________________

3. A flat, folded paper container ________________

4. Computer-to-computer communication ________________

5. Formatted in block and modified block styles ________________

6. A written, printed form of communication to someone in another organization. ________________

7. A summary and record of events and decisions that occur at a meeting ________________

8. A written message to someone in the same organization ________________

9. An instrument by means of which the voice is transmitted to other locations ________________

10. All lines are aligned at the left margin ________________

Writing Exercises

1. The pathologist at LeClaire Hospital needs to send a pathology record on a patient, Mary Anderson, to Dr. Sarah Archie's office at Villes Medical Center across town. Specify which forms are necessary to complete this task.

2. Write a memo to the medical office staff including the information: a meeting October 1, 20XX, at 9:00 a.m. in the conference room for two reasons. The first is how to access records more quickly; the second is to make suggestions on how to use the extra office space.

3. Write the minutes of what took place at the meeting described in exercise 2.

4. Write a letter in block style to Dr. Valerie Christopher. Ask her if she will be a keynote speaker at the New England Medical Conference in Boston on February 8, 20XX. Include information about the title and length of the talk, overnight accommodations, and financial reimbursement.

5. Fill out a phone message form with the necessary information to reflect a call to Dr. Christopher at the Villes Medical Center from Cathy Lizz, Ph.D.

Circle the correctly spelled word in each line:

1. consientious	conshientious	conscientous	conscientious
2. vacination	vaccinition	vaccination	vaccinasion
3. phlegm	phlenm	flgem	phlem
4. personel	personnel	pirsonnel	persunel
5. recupperation	recooperation	recouperation	recuperation
6. jondice	jandice	jaundice	jaundise
7. recomendations	recommendations	recomenditions	recomendashuns
8. indispensible	indispensable	indispencible	indispensble
9. skedule	schedule	skeduuile	schedoul
10. peripheral	perepheral	perpheral	paripheral

Translate medical abbreviations using a medical dictionary or appendix.

1. GTT ____________________
2. °C ____________________
3. ± ____________________
4. = ____________________
5. H/A ____________________
6. TPR ____________________
7. gr ____________________
8. ml ____________________
9. mm ____________________
10. MMR ____________________

Chapter 13

Charting and Documenting

Objectives

Upon completion of this chapter, the student should be able to:

- understand the medical language of abbreviations and symbols
- recognize the different styles of charting in the medical record
- understand the purposes of the medical record
- spell various medical terms
- translate various medical abbreviations and symbols

To provide the continuity essential to quality patient care, there must be a cohesive method in which information is passed on and shared by physicians and other supportive staff. Documentation is that method. Charting and documenting are the instruments that hold the medical team accountable and responsible for the type of services rendered to patients. They are written proof that something was done. The rapid changes in the health-care industry require that accurate, detailed documentation by multilevel personnel involved in the care of patients be maintained at all times. Documentation provides critical evidence regarding patients' reactions, treatment, symptoms, tests, procedures, patient education, medications, and other vital information. Data obtained from documentation are used for diagnosing and assessing a patient's condition.

The Medical Record

The medical record is the specific instrument of documentation that stores written information about a patient's health condition. It is also called the *clinical record* or *medical chart.* One purpose for the medical record is to contain all necessary information needed to provide quality patient care. It provides the evidence that the patient has received treatments, procedures, the medications, and contains other vital information. For example, if a patient is allergic to penicillin and the medical record does not include this critical information, there could be a disaster. Should the patient be given penicillin, it could result in an anaphylactic shock that could be fatal. This simple illustration reflects the importance of documenting and charting medical information. Continuous and up-to-date documentation is vital for proper diagnoses and quality care.

The medical record may be used to gather statistical information for the research and evaluation of certain diseases. Two examples of this are knowing how many pertusis (whooping cough) cases are found in certain geographic areas or understanding the effects of cholesterol on the arteries. Analysis of data found in medical records often leads to better health care, choices of medications, medical procedures, or other important health decisions.

Another important use for the medical record is that it serves as a legal validation of patient care that insurance companies may need to substantiate claims. Attorneys may also access the record for litigation purposes.

In 1928, the American Medical Record Association (AMRA) was founded to improve the standards of documentation. In the early days of medical documentation, the patient's record consisted of one liners that gave very little information. Today, the medical record is a complex file of multiform documents. Some types of information found in medical records are:

patient demographic information	consent for treatment	plan for care
past and current diagnoses	medications	consultation reports
history and physical	dietary restrictions	doctors' orders
known allergies	laboratory tests	radiology reports
hospital discharge summaries	treatments	progress notes

The Joint commission on Accreditation of Healthcare Organizations (JCAHO) has the responsibility of accrediting health-care facilities. In order to achieve accreditation status, a facility's medical records must meet certain standards regarding entries, types of information documented, formats, correction procedures, abbreviations and symbols, completeness of data, timely recordings, dates, deadlines, signatures, and various other legal documents.

State and local laws govern the retention of medical records. Some physicians keep them for an indefinite period of time. The physician or the facility owns the physical record itself. The patient owns the information in the medical record. For this reason, health personnel are responsible for safeguarding the confidentiality of the patient. Many employees are required to sign a confidentiality statement.

Certain features are essential when charting data in medical records. They include the following:

Documentation	Only authorized individuals are responsible for documenting patient care. The record must contain all original reports.
Signature	Professionals must sign entries and reports to verify that care is given. Rules and regulations govern this area.
Abbreviations	Only approved medical abbreviations and symbols must be used.
Timeliness	All entries should be written as soon as possible.
Legibility	Records need to be legible. If possible, reports should be typed.
Accuracy	A mistake in an entry is corrected by drawing a single line through the error and writing the correction above it. The entry must be initialed and dated. Correction fluid is *never* used.
Writing Style	Entries into the medical record must be brief, accurate, and to the point.
Organization	Organization of medical records promotes efficiency and accuracy. Physicians and specialists usually select the organizational style of the medical record. A specialist who sees a patient occasionally will not need complex records. A specialist who sees a patient frequently needs a detailed format.

> *Accurate and well-documented medical records are necessary if the medical office is to run smoothly.*

Appropriate documentation is very critical in medical records. If done incorrectly, it can have legal ramifications. Consider these rules:

1. Use short, accurate phrases and sentences.
2. If there is a space left blank, draw a line through it so no one can write in the space.
3. Proofread all entries.
4. Never use correction fluid to fix errors.
5. Never document before the fact.
6. Only use approved abbreviations.
7. Be absolutely sure you have the correct chart before writing.
8. State facts.
9. Record the date and time of entry.

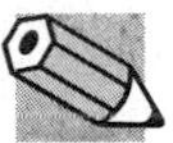

Practice 13-1

Respond to these items:

1. State three purposes for the medical record.

___

___

___

2. Name four items found in the medical record.

___

___

___

___

3. What is the meaning of JCAHO?

___

4. Who owns the information in the medical record?

___

5. Documenting and charting includes all of the following except ________________

   a. patient's reaction to procedures   c. insurance bills

   b. medications   d. tests

Answer true or false to these statements:

1. Opinions may be added to the medical record. _____
2. The American Medical Association (AMA) provides accreditation to medical facilities. _____
3. The medical record is a legal document. _____
4. Sentences but not phrases are used in the medical record. _____

The Language of the Medical Record

The use of abbreviations is a standard practice in charting, reporting, and documenting medical information. They form the background and essence of the medical language and originate from a variety of sources.

Examples

Observation regarding a patient's condition:

Pt appears cyanotic.

Pt. appears anxious and apprehensive.

Documenting assistance in physiological functions:

Pt. I&O was recorded.

Pt. ↑ ambulation today.

Documenting assistance with pain or comfort measures:

Pt was given pain meds.

Pt. given lamb's wool for comfort.

Documenting written or verbal orders:

Doctor ordered Pt. OOB t.i.d.

Dr. ordered P.T. q. day.

General Rules for Abbreviations

Abbreviations and acronyms are used often in the medical field. They are the shorthand of the medical profession. Abbreviations may contain both upper- and lowercase letters and may or may not take periods. Here are some general rules:

- Educational degrees are abbreviated and punctuated: M.D., Ph.D., D.D.S., M. Ed., B.A.
- Certification and registrations do not have to be punctuated with periods: RN, CAGS, CMA, CMT
- Acronyms are capitalized and follow their formal name:

  AIDS, Acquired Immunodeficiency Syndrome

  POMR, Problem-oriented medical record

  PERRLA, pupils, equal, regular, react to light and accommodation
- Abbreviations are used in chart notes, but not in formal correspondence:

  Chart note: *Pt* is to have a *FBS* in the *a.m.*

  Formal correspondence: The patient is to have a fasting blood sugar test in the morning.
- Chemical abbreviations use upper- and lowercase letters: KCI, K, Na
- Do not use the same courtesy title at the beginning and end of a name:

  Incorrect Dr. Chris Villmare, M.D.

  Correct Chris Villmare, M.D. or Dr. Chris Villmare
- Do not abbreviate the days of the week or the months of the year:

  Incorrect Feb. 18, 1999 2-18-2006 2-18-2020

  Correct February 18, 2006
- Latin abbreviations are usually in lowercase letters: i.e., a.c., p.m., a.m., o.d., a.u.
- Measurements are abbreviated without using a period: cm, 500 mg, 30 ml, 30 cc
- A comma is not necessary when II or III follows a surname: John Archie III
- Abbreviations are acceptable in formal reports, as long as the word was spelled out previously.
- Spell out diagnoses and procedures to prevent misinterpretations: Marshall-Marchetti operation, tonsillectomy and adenoidectomy
- Symbols are acceptable as a shortened form of communication: 4-0 silk suture, 56% bone loss, 2+
- All abbreviations and symbols must be accepted and approved by the medical staff for use at a particular facility.
- In medical correspondence, use the two letter abbreviations (without periods) for the states:

  Alabama, AL
  Alaska, AK
  Arizona, AZ
  Arkansas, AR
  California, CA
  Colorado, CO
  Connecticut, CT
  Delaware, DE
  District of Columbia, DC
  Florida, FL
  Georgia, GA
  Hawaii, HI
  Idaho, ID
  Illinois, IL
  Indiana, IN
  Iowa, IA
  Kansas, KS
  Kentucky, KY
  Louisiana, LA
  Maine, ME
  Maryland, MD
  Massachusetts, MA
  Michigan, MI
  Minnesota, MN
  Mississippi, MS
  Missouri, MO
  Montana, MT
  Nebraska, NE
  Nevada, NV
  New Hampshire, NH
  New Jersey, NJ
  New Mexico, NM

New York, NY
North Carolina, NC
North Dakota, ND
Ohio, OH
Oklahoma, OK
Oregon, OR
Pennsylvania, PA
Rhode Island, RI
South Carolina, SC
South Dakota, SD
Tennessee, TN
Texas, TX
Utah, UT
Vermont, VT
Virginia, VA
Washington, WA
West Virginia, WV
Wisconsin, WI
Wyoming, WY

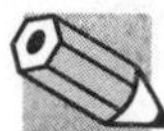

Practice 13-2

Select the correct form from each pair:

1.	Dr. William LeClaire, M.D.	Dr. William LeClaire
2.	Jan. 8, 20XX	January 8, 20XX
3.	9:15 a.m.	9:15 A.M.
4.	American Medical Association (AMA)	(AMA) American Medical Association
5.	Valerie Villmare, CMA	Valerie Villmare, C.M.A.
6.	Chris Villmare, II	Chris Villmare II
7.	3 cm.	3 cm
8.	Chicago, IL	Chicago, IN
9.	Boston, MA	Boston, MA.
10.	98%	98 percent

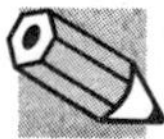

Practice 13-3

Translate these abbreviations:

1. Htn __________________
2. HR __________________
3. o.u. __________________
4. pre op __________________
5. IBD __________________
6. a.d. __________________

7. ASA ____________________

8. meds. ____________________

9. AAMA ____________________

10. CHF ____________________

11. lytes ____________________

12. BP ____________________

13. DOB ____________________

14. h.s. ____________________

15. BRP ____________________

16. CA ____________________

17. noc ____________________

18. CABG ____________________

19. CAD ____________________

20. D&C ____________________

Common Types of Charting

There are many types of charting. The method for your facility is the method that should be followed. Many institutions develop a combination of types of charting.

Traditional or Narrative Charting

Narrative notes are phrases, clauses, and sentences without any specific structure. They are traditional notes that were used for many years and were lengthy, containing both important and unimportant information such as "pt. is comfortable, visitors today." For many years the narrative notes were thrown away after a patient was discharged and not kept as part of the permanent record.

Through the years, many factors motivated the need for changes in written documentation: legal requirements, Medicare reimbursement, insurance benefits, billing and coding practices, to name just a few reasons.

Because people perceive and interpret information differently, it was difficult to streamline charting and documenting. Concise and focused charting has been developed in more recent times. Today, narrative charting communicates only essential facts about the patient.

Example

5-30-20XX 9 pm Pt. c/o pain over the incision. Pain med administered. Pt. voided 150cc 5 hrs. after Foley cath was removed.

11pm Pt still c/o pain. Dr. Villes notified.

D. Oberg, R.N.

5-30-20XX 12midnoc Dr. Villes in to examine pt. Increased dosage of pain med.

L. Villmare, CMA

This type of information is often placed in the source-oriented medical record (SOMR). It is a simple system and requires the least amount of work and organization.

SOAP

Lawrence Weed, M.D., instituted the problem-oriented medical record (POMR) method in 1969, at Case Western Reserve in Cleveland. The POMR organizes the patient's record in a comprehensive manner by charting the patient's problems in order of importance and how those problems are addressed. Some institutions still use this format. Others have incorporated part of the format to fit their own charting and documenting needs. POMR has four parts:

1. *Data base.* The data consists of information from various sources that identifies the problem and is the basis for evaluating the patient's health.
2. *Problem list.* This is a chronological list of the patient's problems and reasons for seeing the doctor.
3. *Initial plan.* A treatment plan is developed to address each problem the patient has.
4. *Progress notes.* The notes written are called subjective-objective-assessment-plan—or SOAP—notes. In this format, progress notes are dated, headed, and numbered for specific problems.

SOAP notes consist of:

S A history and *subjective* data told to the physician by the patient or a family member; such as nausea, descriptions of symptoms, and feeling.

Examples

I have a pain in my leg.

pt. c/o pain in the lower back.

pt. c/o migraine headache.

O Objective data from the physician's physical exam of what is seen, heard, and touched.

Examples

results from tests and physical exam.

weeping, inflammation, vital signs.

If, for instance, a patient comes to the ER and is complaining of being hot, and is perspiring and flushed, the entry might read like this:

S—Pt. complains of temperature and diaphoresis.

O—V.S. taken: T-102 , P-80, R-24, B.P. 150/80, diaphoretic

A An assessment by the physician with diagnoses and impressions.

Examples

arthritis of the leg

Dx: *emphysema*

pt. has chronic bronchiolitis

P A treatment plan for medical problems, medications, consults, surgery, and patient education.

Examples

Take ASA q. 4 h. for pain

Pt. to PT 3 X wk.

SOAPE

SOAP notes were later modified to include evaluation:

E An evaluation stating how the patient responded to the illness and reacted to the treatment, medications, and medical care.

SOAPIE

Another system added intervention and its evaluation:

I An intervention is an approach to a particular problem.
E The evaluation looks at the response of the intervention in terms of the illness and subsequent treatment.

Figure 13-1 is an example of SOAPIE charting.

SOAPIER

Other components to the SOAP system of charting include intervention, evaluation, and revision.

I Intervention considers the approach to a particular problem.
E Evaluation looks at the patient's response to the treatment intervention.
R Revision identifies changes that are prompted by the evaluation.

PIE

Problem-intervention-evaluation (PIE) charting was introduced in 1984 at the Craven Regional Medical Center in North Carolina. With this method, problems are identified and addressed at least once on every shift. Teaching plans are incorporated in the progress notes. Notes must be read often to understand the evolution of the problems and the effectiveness of the treatment.

Examples

P Problem: *Pt hasn't had BM for 3 days.*

Nurse's Progress Record

Date	Hour	Progress Notes
10/14/01	0730	Problem #2 Ketoacidosis S: Client states "I feel sick all over." Client claims difficulty in breathing, abdominal pain + nausea. O: Lungs clear, R 28/min, labored. Abdomen distended, bowel sounds underactive all 4 quadrants. Abdominal pain 5 on a 0-10 pain scale. A: Alteration in nutrition + comfort R/T ketoacidosis. Blood glucose 458 mg/dl. Ketones strongly positive. pH < 7.3. P: Maintain IV infusion of 0.9% NS c̄ regular insulin as ordered. NPO. Oral hygiene hrly. Maintain accurate I+O. Assess for rales, hypotension, cardiac dysrhythmias. Monitor blood glucose electrolytes. — L. White RN
10/14/01	0730	I: Called Dr. Singh, blood glucose 458 mg/dl IV bolus regular insulin given as ordered. 1000 ml 0.9% N.S. infusing @ 1 l/H central line #1 via infusion pump. 50 u regular insulin in 500 ml N.S. infusing @ 50 ml/H central line #2 via infusion pump. EKG taken, placed on telemetry.
10/14/01	0835	E: Lungs clear, R 24/min, non-labored. NSR abdominal pain 3 on a 0-10 pain scale. Urinary output 750 ml/hr. Blood glucose 360 mg/dl. — L. White RN

Figure 13-1 Sample SOAPIE Charting

I Intervention: *T.O. for MOM 30 ml. 8am*

E Evaluation: *Pt. had a BM in afternoon.*

Figure 13-2 is an example of PIE charting.

An office may use SOAP notes, traditional narrative charting, or other types of charting. Medical offices, hospitals, and clinics usually develop their own methods of charting that best accommodate their particular situations. Data such as test results, abbreviations, and medical reports usually remain the same, but the organization of the documentation is unique to each locale. In any event, the ultimate goal of organizing documentation is to provide easier access to patient information, particularly in today's medical environment where so many different professionals access medical records.

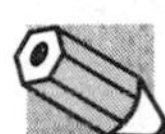

Practice 13-4

Translate the following abbreviations and determine if the statement is subjective. Consult the abbreviation list.

1. Pt. c/o SOB ____________________
2. Check I & O q. h. ____________________
3. Dx: URI ____________________
4. OOB adlib post op ____________________
5. U/A for RBC ____________________
6. D/C Coumadin STAT ____________________

Respond to the following items:

1. The term STAT means ____________________.

   a. immediately b. by mouth c. whenever necessary d. stand by

2. An example of subjective information is ____________________.

   a. giving pain medication b. a patient's complaint

   c. history of the problem d. physical therapy

3. Dr. Lawrence Weed developed a medical record system called ____________________.

   a. HMRO b. the raditional method

   c. POMR d. chronological system

4. Which of the following is subjective?

   a. diagnosis b. treatment c. lab report d. past surgical history

Nurse's Progress Record

Date	Hour	Progress Notes
10/14/01	0730	**P:** altered nutrition R/T ketoacidosis. Blood glucose 458mg/dl. ketones strongly positive, pH 7.2.
		I: called Dr. Singh, blood glucose 458mg/dl IV bolus regular insulin given as ordered. 1000ml 0.9% N.S. infusing @ 1L/H central line #1 via infusion pump. 50u regular insulin in 500 ml N.S. infusing @50ml/H, central line #2 via infusion pump. EKG taken, placed on telemetry.
10/14/01	0835	**E:** Lungs clear, R 24/min nonlabored. NSR, abdominal pain 3 on a 0-10 pain scale. Urinary output 750 ml/H (0730-0830) Blood sugar 320mg/dl. — L. White RN —

Figure 13-2 Sample PIE Charting

Medical Spelling

Become familiar with the spelling of the following words:

assessment
cachexia
carcinogens
chemotherapeutic
cytology
dehiscence
dementia
diabetes
diffusion
dysplasia
emesis
endogenous
endoscopy
enteric
episodic
evisceration
exacerbation
fissure
fluoroscopy
immunoglobulins
incontinence
influenza
insomnia
integrity
interferon
interstitial
intoxication
manifestation
mediastinum
narcolepsy
neurophysiologic
oxygenation
pathophysiology
pediculosis
perceptual
pericarditis
rehabilitation
stenosis
syndrome
tolerance
ultrasound
vertilligo
visceral

Charting and Documenting Study Summary

The Medical Record	Specific instruments of documentation that store written information about a patient's health condition.
Language of the Medical Record	Use medical terms and abbreviations for documenting medical information.

General Rules for Abbreviations:

Abbreviate acronyms—AIDS

Abbreviate chart notes

Abbreviate chemical symbols

Use lower case letters in Latin abbreviations

Measurement abbreviations have no periods

Abbreviations are acceptable in formal reports if previously spelled out—tonsillectomy and adenoidectomy: T&A

States have two letter abbreviations—MA, NY

Certifications and registrations have no periods—RN, CMT, CMA

In formal writing, days of the week and months of the year are not abbreviated—February 18, 20XX

A comma is not necessary when II or III follow a surname—John Archie IV

Types of charting

Traditional	A type of charting that uses phrases, clauses, and sentences without any specific structure.
Problem Oriented Medical Record (POMR)	Charting problems by order of importance.
SOAP	An acronym meaning:
	S—subjective data: feelings and description of symptoms.
	O—objective data: data from physical exam.
	A—assessment: diagnosis and impressions.
	P—plan: medication, treatments, consults, surgery
SOAPE	E—evaluation: patient's response to treatment
SOAPIE	I—intervention: an approach to a particular problem.
	E—evaluating that approach.
SOAPIER	I—intervention: approach to a problem
	E—evaluating that approach
	R—revision: changes prompted by the evaluation.
PIE	Problem—Intervention: Evaluation
	Problems are identified and addressed at least once on every shift.

Skills Review

Translate these abbreviations and symbols using a medical dictionary or appendix.

1. SC ____________________
2. SGPT ____________________
3. TB ____________________
4. ad lib ____________________
5. po ____________________
6. ADH ____________________
7. a.u. ____________________
8. BMR ____________________

9. BS ________________

10. IV ________________

11. ECHO ________________

12. RBC ________________

13. TPR ________________

14. ROS ________________

15. ESR ________________

16. WBC ________________

17. ELISA ________________

18. GERD ________________

19. GI ________________

20. ⇌ ________________

21. LUL ________________

22. Bx ________________

23. VS ________________

24. IDDM ________________

25. TIA ________________

26. ↓ ________________

27. // ________________

28. soln ________________

29. US ________________

30. O.D. ________________

31. PE ________________

32. PPD ________________

33. || ____________________

34. EKG ____________________

35. ℞ ____________________

36. HEENT ____________________

Write either S for subjective, O for objective, or N if neither:

1. Pt. c/o pain in the epigastric region ____________________
2. H&H lower this wk ____________________
3. TIA ten yrs ago ____________________
4. Dx: COLD ____________________
5. States Hx of COPD ____________________
6. C/O ↓ back pain ____________________
7. Referred to HEENT for a workup ____________________
8. ↑ pain when walking ____________________
9. ↓ pain with rest ____________________
10. P.E. was WNL ____________________

Translate the following and label O only if the statement is objective information:

1. Pt. to go to P.T. via wheelchair q.o.d. ____________________
2. Pt. appears cyanotic. ____________________
3. Apply ice to the ankle for 24 hrs. ____________________
4. T- 101° F ____________________
5. Pt. c/o sore throat. ____________________
6. Right ankle swollen ____________________
7. BM x 4 in a.m. ____________________
8. ROM is WNL ____________________
9. CBC results in the chart. ____________________
10. Rx: Hot packs to both knees q.i.d. ____________________

Circle the correctly spelled word in each line:

1 chemotherputic	chemotherapeutic	chemotheraputic	chemotherapuetic
2. dihiscence	dehiscence	dehisence	dehissence
3. evisceration	evicseration	evisserration	eviseraetion
4. difusion	diffussion	diffusion	difuesion
5. intoxcication	intoxsication	intoxecation	intoxication
6. narcopsy	narrcolepsy	narkolepsy	narcolepsy
7. dysplasia	dyspaysia	dysplaysia	displasia
8. imunoglobulins	inmunoglobulins	immunoglobulins	immunoglobbulins
9. incontenence	incontinence	incontanence	incontonance
10. asessment	asesment	assessment	assesment

Translate the following information and label it S (subjective) or O (objective) only if either label applies:

1. Father stated that the son had an appendectomy 3 years ago. ________________
2. D/C meds ________________
3. 3 gtts A.U. q.i.d. ________________
4. Hx of ASHD and Htn ________________
5. Pt. denies pain with coughing. ________________
6. Dx is otitis media ________________
7. Pt. c/o urticaria and itching ________________
8. B.P. 160/100 ________________
9. Place Pt. in Fowler's position for better breathing. ________________
10. Vertigo ________________

Identify the meaning of these phrases:

1. Record I&O x 3 d. ________________

2. 3 gtt a.u. q.d. ____________________

3. Dx: URI ____________________

4. FBS on adm. ____________________

5. U/A for RBC's ____________________

Write the symbol for these words:

1. greater than ____________________

2. tablet ____________________

3. male ____________________

4. primary ____________________

5. right ____________________

6. left ____________________

7. without ____________________

8. of each ____________________

9. approximately ____________________

10. before ____________________

Chapter 14

Introduction to Medical Reports

Objectives

Upon completion of this chapter, the student should be able to:

- recognize the various kinds of medical reports
- identify the content of each report
- spell various medical terms
- translate various medical abbreviations and symbols

History and Physical

A history and physical (H&P) report is usually dictated after a new patient is admitted to a hospital or comes to a clinic, office, or health facility. The H&P is a collection of data about past events in relation to a patient's present illness. Its purpose is to aid in understanding the whole patient, past and present, in order to form a treatment plan based on how the patient can be helped in the future.

The format of the report varies from place to place and is usually generated by the medical facility's Form Committee. Regardless of the format, however, the type of information sought is universal.

The historical component is an account of the patient's systems and organs based on information rooted in the past, such as family and social histories, previous hospitalizations or treatments, allergies, chronic illness, and the patient's chief complaints. The physical component of the H&P is not historical. It is the physician's current evaluation of the patient's systems and organs.

A sample H&P follows:

HISTORY AND PHYSICAL EXAMINATION (H&P)

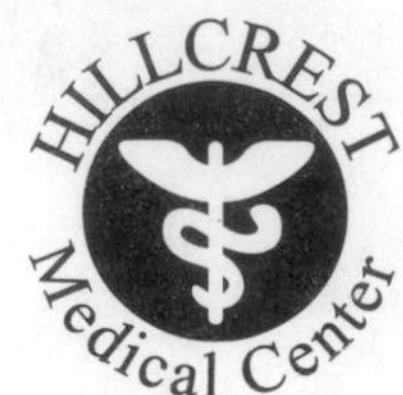

Patient Name: Roger Parks

Hospital No.: 11009

Room No.: 812

Date of Admission: 12/01/20XX

Admitting Physician: Steven Benard, M.D.

Admitting Diagnosis: Rule out appendicitis.

CHIEF COMPLAINT: Abdominal pain.

HISTORY OF PRESENT ILLNESS: The patient is a 31-year-old white man with acute onset of right lower quadrant pain waking him up from sleep at approximately 3 a.m. on the morning of admission. The pain worsened throughout the day, radiating to his back and becoming associated with dry heaves. The patient states that the pain is constant and is worsened by walking or movement. The patient states his last bowel movement was on the previous evening and was normal. The patient is anorectic. He also gives a 1-year history of lower abdominal colicky pain associated with diarrhea. He was seen by his local medical doctor and given a diagnosis of irritable bowel syndrome; however, the pain is worse tonight and is unlike his previous bouts of abdominal pain. The patient also has had associated fever and chills to date.

PAST HISTORY: SURGICAL: No previous operations.
ILLNESSES: None. Hospitalization for epididymitis 10 years ago. He is ALLERGIC TO PENICILLIN. It makes him bloated. MEDICATIONS: None.

SOCIAL HISTORY: Carpenter. Lives with his wife and two children. He does not drink or smoke.

FAMILY HISTORY: Insignificant for familial inflammatory bowel disease except for the fact that his mother has colonic polyps. Father living and well. No siblings.

REVIEW OF SYSTEMS: Noncontributory.

PHYSICAL EXAMINATION: This is a 31-year-old white man with knees raised to his abdomen and complaining of severe pain. VITAL SIGNS: Admission temperature 99.6F; four hours after admission it was 102.6F. HEENT: Normocephalic, atraumatic, EOMs intact, negative icterus, conjunctivae pink. NECK: Supple. No adenopathy or bruits noted. CHEST: Clear to auscultation and percussion. CARDIAC: Regular rate and rhythm. No murmurs noted. Peripheral pulses 2+ and symmetrical. ABDOMEN: Bowel sounds initially positive but diminished. He has positive cough reflex, positive heel tap, and positive rebound tenderness. The pain is definitely worse in his RLQ. RECTAL: Heme negative. Tenderness toward the RLQ. Normal prostate. Normal male genitalia. EXTREMITIES: No clubbing, cyanosis, or edema. NEUROLOGIC: Nonfocal.

(*Continued*)

HISTORY AND PHYSICAL EXAMINATION
Patient Name: Roger Parks
Hospital No.: 11009
Page 2

LABORATORY DATA: Hemoglobin 14.6, hematocrit 43.6, and 13,000 WBCs. Sodium 138, potassium 3.8, chloride 105, CO_2 24, BUN 10, creatinine 0.9, and glucose 102. Amylase was 30. UA completely negative. LFTs within normal limits. Alkaline phosphatase 78, GGT 9, SGOT 39, GPT 12, bilirubin 0.9. Flat plate and upright films of the abdomen revealed localized abnormal gas pattern in right lower quadrant. No evidence of free air.

ASSESSMENT: Rule out appendicitis. Some concern of whether this could be an exacerbation of developing inflammatory bowel disease. Due to the patient's history, increasing temperature, and localizing symptoms to his right lower quadrant, the patient needs surgical intervention to rule out appendicitis.

Steven Benard, M.D.

SB:xx
D:12/01/20XX
T:12/01/20XX

M.A. Novak and P.A. Ireland, *Hillcrest Medical Center Beginning Medical Transcription Course,* 5th ed. Albany, NY: Delmar Thomson Learning, 1999, pp. 19–20.

Consultation Report

When a consultation has been requested to obtain a second opinion on a problem or diagnosis, a consultation report is prepared for the referring physician. It contains such data as present medical history, x-ray and lab results, and the consulted physician's impressions, recommendations, evaluations, diagnoses, and treatment.

Promptness in providing information is very important. The consultation report format may be a letter or a specially prepared form with the date and reason for consultation. It is also proper to include a thank you for the referral. The report is dictated by the consulting physician and transcribed in the medical office or through outside services.

A sample consultation report follows:

REQUEST FOR CONSULTATION

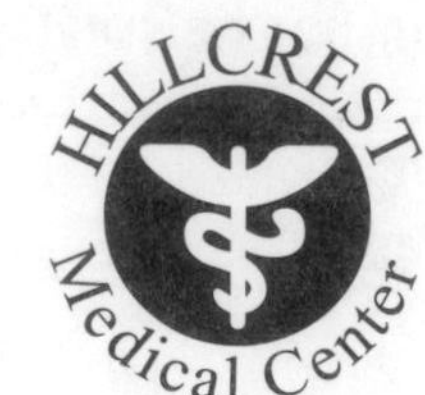

Patient Name: Marty Gibbs

Hospital No.: 11532

Consultant: Patrick O'Neill, M.D., Plastic Surgery

Requesting Physician: Diane Houston, M.D., Internal Medicine

Date: 11/25/20XX

Reason for Consultation: Please evaluate extent of burn injuries.

BURNING AGENT: Coals in fire pit.

I have been asked to see this 5-year-old Caucasian male who appears in mild distress due to upper extremity burn after having fallen into hot coals in his back yard.

Using the Lund Browder chart,[4] the severity of burn is first and second degree. The total body surface area burned includes right lower arm 3%, right hand 1%. The joints involved include the right elbow, right wrist, right hand.

TREATMENT PLAN: Splinting right hand.
Positioning: Elevation with splint on.
Range of motion: Good mobility.
Pressure therapy: Will follow for induration, for pressure fracture.

GOALS:
1. Reduce risk of contractures of involved joints by positioning, splinting, and maintaining range of motion.
2. Reduce scar tissue formation by using Jobst bandages, pressure therapy, and splinting.
3. Obtain maximum mobility and strength of upper extremities.
4. Maximize independence in activities of daily living. Activity as tolerated.
5. Provide patient and family education regarding high-calorie, high-protein diet.

(*Continued*)

[4]See page 221: The Lund Browder Chart.

REQUEST FOR CONSULTATION
Patient Name: Marty Gibbs
Hospital No.: 11532
Page 2

Thank you for asking me to see this delightful boy. I will follow him at the burn clinic in 2 weeks.

Patrick O'Neill, M.D.

PO:xx
D:11/25/20XX
T:11/28/20XX

M.A. Novak and P.A. Ireland, *Hillcrest Medical Center Beginning Medical Transcription Course,* 5th ed. Albany, NY: Delmar Thomson Learning, 1999, pp. 26–27.

Radiology Report

A radiology report describes the results of a diagnostic procedure using radio waves or other forms of radiation. Examples of such procedures are x-rays, CT scans, MRI, upper GI series, and ultrasonogram. Medical words ending in *scopy* or *graphy* usually involve radiologic procedures. These medical procedures provide visual images to aid in diagnosis. A *radiologist* is the physician who interprets the images and provides the radiology report.

A sample radiology report follows:

RADIOLOGY REPORT

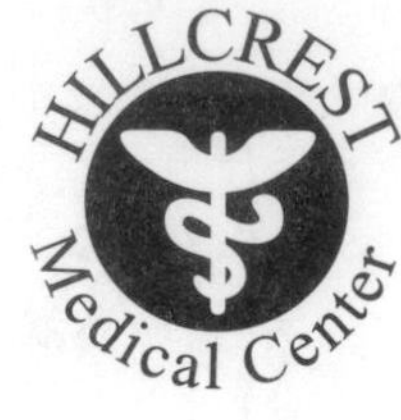

Patient Name: Marietta Mosley

Hospital No.: 11446

X-ray No.: 98-2801

Admitting Physician: John Youngblood, M.D.

Procedure: Left hip x-ray.

Date: 08/05/20XX

PRIMARY DIAGNOSIS: Fractured left hip.

CLINICAL INFORMATION: Left hip pain. No known allergies.

Orthopedic device is noted transfixing the left femoral neck. I have no old films available for comparison. The left femoral neck region appears anatomically aligned. At the level of an orthopedic screw along the lateral aspect of the femoral neck, approximately at the level of the lesser trochanter, there is a radiolucent band consistent with a fracture of indeterminate age that shows probable nonunion. There is bilateral marginal sclerosis and moderate offset and angulation at this site.

Fairly exuberant callus formation is noted laterally along the femoral shaft.

IMPRESSION:

1. No evidence for significant displacement at the femoral neck.
2. Probable nonunion of fracture transversely through the shaft of the femur at about the level of the lesser trochanter.

Neil Nofsinger, M.D.

NN:xx
D:08/05/20XX
T:08/05/20XX

M.A. Novak and P.A. Ireland, *Hillcrest Medical Center Beginning Medical Transcription Course,* 5th ed. Albany, NY: Delmar Thomson Learning, 1999, p. 21.

Pathology Report

A pathology report contains a description of tissue samples removed from the body. The removal of a tissue sample for examination is called a *biopsy.* The *pathologist* is the person who studies the tissue samples and generates the pathology report.

The focus of the pathology report is twofold:

1. Macroscopic findings (also called Gross Description, Gross Examination). This component describes how the specimen looks to the naked eye. It describes the size, general color, and texture.
2. Microscopic findings (also called Microscopic Description). This component describes how tissue looks when examined under a microscope.

The report usually ends with a diagnosis of the findings or an impression.

The pathology report is the examination of specific tissues. The pathology report becomes a permanent part of the patient's medical record. A sample pathology report is provided on page 276.

Discharge Summary

The discharge summary is a report that is required for all patients that leave the health-care facility. It is a summary of the patient's condition during his or her stay at the facility. Data in the discharge summary include:

- Reason for admittance
- History of present illness
- Social history
- Physical exam and laboratory data
- Events that occurred during the patient's stay
- Follow-up instructions
- Discharge medications

The report concludes with the condition of the patient at the time of discharge and the discharge prognosis. A sample discharge summary follows on page 277.

PATHOLOGY REPORT

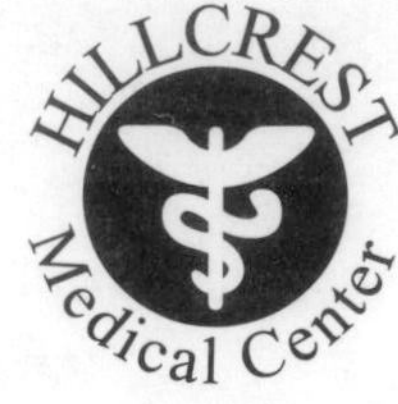

Patient Name: Sumio Yukimura

Hospital No.: 11449

Pathology Report No.: 98-S-942

Admitting Physician: Donna Yates, M.D.

Preoperative Diagnosis: Cholelithiasis.

Postoperative Diagnosis: Cholelithiasis.

Specimen Submitted: Gallbladder and stone.

Date Received: 06/05/20XX

Date Reported: 06/06/20XX

GROSS DESCRIPTION: Specimen received in one container labeled "gallbladder." Specimen consists of a 9-cm gallbladder measuring 2 cm in average diameter. The serosal surface demonstrates diffuse fibrous adhesion. The wall is thickened and hemorrhagic. The mucosa is eroded, and there is a single large stone measuring 2 cm in diameter within the lumen. Representative sections are submitted in one cassette.

GROSS DIAGNOSIS: Gallstone.

KM:xx
D:06/05/20XX
T:06/05/20XX

MICROSCOPIC DIAGNOSIS: Gallbladder, hemorrhagic chronic cholecystitis with cholelithiasis.

Robert Thompson, M.D.

RT:xx
D:06/06/20XX
T:06/06/20XX

M.A. Novak and P.A. Ireland, *Hillcrest Medical Center Beginning Medical Transcription Course,* 5th ed. Albany, NY: Delmar Thomson Learning, 1999, p. 23.

DISCHARGE SUMMARY

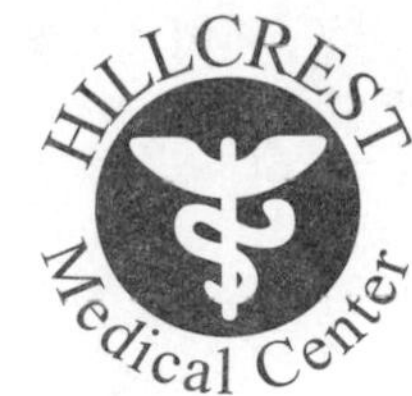

Patient Name: Joyce Mabry

Hospital No.: 11709

Admitted: 02/18/20XX

Discharged: 02/24/20XX

Consultations: Tom Moore, M.D., Hematology

Procedures: Splenectomy.

Complications: None.

Admitting Diagnosis: Elective splenectomy for idiopathic thrombocytopenic purpura and systemic lupus erythematosus.

HISTORY: The patient is a 21-year-old white woman who had noted excessive bruising since last June. She was diagnosed as having thrombocytopenic purpura. At the same time, the diagnosis of systemic lupus erythematosus was made. The patient continues with the bruising. The patient had been treated with steroids, prednisone 20 mg; however, the platelet count has remained low, less than 20,000. The patient was admitted for elective splenectomy.

LABORATORY DATA ON ADMISSION: Chest x-ray was negative. Electrocardiogram was normal. Sodium 138, potassium 5.2, chloride 104, CO_2 25, glucose 111. Urinalysis negative. Hemoglobin 14.8, hematocrit 43.5, white blood cell count 15,000, platelet count 17,000, PT 11.5, PTT 27.

HOSPITAL COURSE: The patient was taken to the operating room on February 19 where a splenectomy was performed. The patient's postoperative course was uncomplicated with the wound healing well. The platelet count was stable for the first 3 postoperative days. The patient was transfused intraoperatively with 10 units of platelets and postoperatively with 10 additional units of platelets. However, on the fourth postoperative day the platelet count had risen to 77,000, which was a significant increase.

The patient was discharged for follow-up in my office. She will also be seen by Dr. Moore, who will follow her SLE and ITP.

DISCHARGE DIAGNOSIS: Idiopathic thrombocytopenic purpura and systemic lupus erythematosus.

(*Continued*)

DISCHARGE SUMMARY
Patient Name: Joyce Mabry
Hospital No.: 11709
Page 2

DISCHARGE MEDICATIONS:
1. Prednisone 20 mg q.d.
2. Percocet 1 to 2 p.o. q. 4 h. p.r.n.
3. Multivitamins, 1 in a.m. q.d.

____
Carmen Garcia, M.D.

CG:xx
D:02/25/20XX
T:02/26/20XX

M.A. Novak and P.A. Ireland, *Hillcrest Medical Center Beginning Medical Transcription Course,* 5th ed. Albany, NY: Delmar Thomson Learning, 1999, pp. 26–27.

Operative Report

The operative report is a comprehensive description of a surgical procedure performed on a patient. The report includes specific details about preoperative, operative, and postoperative experiences such as specimens removed and sent to pathology, diagnosis, type of operation performed, names of surgeons and assistants present, type of anesthesia, instruments used, drain packs, closure, sponge count, suture materials and thickness, any unusual circumstances or complications, and estimated blood loss.

The report may be in narrative form or divided into subheadings, such as "anesthesia," "incision," "findings," "procedures," and "closing." The report details end with the patient going to the recovery room. The operative report must be dictated and filed in medical records as soon as possible after surgery. A sample operative report follows:

OPERATIVE REPORT

HILLCREST Medical Center

Patient Name: Kathy Sullivan

Hospital No.: 11525

Date of Surgery: 06/25/20XX

Admitting Physician: Taylor Withers, M.D.

Surgeons: Sang Lee, M.D., Taylor Withers, M.D.

Preoperative Diagnosis: Urinary incontinence secondary to cystourethrocele.

Postoperative Diagnosis: Urinary incontinence secondary to cystourethrocele.

Operative Procedure: Total abdominal hysterectomy with Marshall-Marchetti correction.

Anesthesia: General endotracheal.

DESCRIPTION: After an abdominal hysterectomy had been performed by Dr. Withers, the peritoneum was closed by him and the procedure was turned over to me.

At this time the supravesical space was entered. The anterior portions of the bladder and urethra were dissected free by blunt and sharp dissection. Bleeders were clamped and electrocoagulated as they were encountered. A wedge of the overlying periosteum was taken and roughened with a bone rasp. The urethra was then attached to the overlying symphysis by placing two No. 1 catgut sutures on each side of the urethra and one in the bladder neck. The urethra and bladder neck pulled up to the overlying symphysis bone very easily with no tension on the sutures. Bleeding was controlled by pulling the bladder neck up to the bone. Penrose drains were placed on each side of the vesical gutter. Blood loss was negligible. The procedure was then turned back over to Dr. Withers, who proceeded with closure.

Sang Lee, M.D.

SL:xx
D:06/25/20XX
T:06/26/20XX

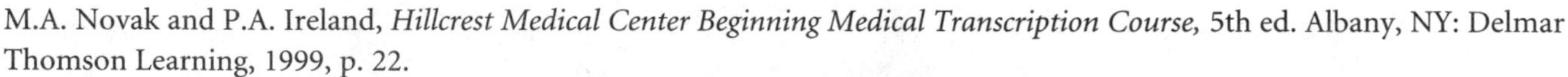

M.A. Novak and P.A. Ireland, *Hillcrest Medical Center Beginning Medical Transcription Course,* 5th ed. Albany, NY: Delmar Thomson Learning, 1999, p. 22.

Medical Spelling

Become familiar with the spelling of the following words:

adipose
agglutination
anemia
anthropometric
antibody
atherosclerosis
atrophy
bilirubin
cardiomyopathy
cerumen
contamination
debridement
dysuria
electrolyte
erythema
erythrocytes
excoriation
fatigue
fluctuation
gait
homeostasis
ischemic
leukemia
leukocytes
malaise
mediastinal
morphology
petechiae
prostheses
radiation
rales
rhonchi
sedimentation
septicemia
thrombocytes
tonsillitis
toxemia
ventilation
wheal
wheeze

Introduction to Medical Reports Study Summary

History and Physical A report containing data about past events in relation to a patient's present illness.

Consultation A report containing data such as present medical history, x-ray, lab results, consulted physician's impressions, recommendations, evaluations, diagnoses, and treatments.

Radiology A report describing the results of a diagnostic procedure using radio waves or other forms of radiation.

Pathology A report containing a description of tissue samples removed from the body.

Discharge Summary A report summarizing the patient's condition while at a healthcare facility.

Operative Report A report describing a surgical procedure performed on a patient.

Skills Review

Use these words to complete the sentences.

macroscopic findings	pathologist	microscopic findings
pathology report	biopsy	discharge summary
follow-up instructions	paramedic	laboratory

1. The part of the pathology report that describes how tissue looks to the naked eye is ____________________.
2. The report that documents what happens during hospitalization is ____________________.
3. The person who examines diseased tissue is a ____________________.
4. A special report that examines the cause of disease is a ____________________.

Circle the correctly spelled word in each line:

1. protsothses	prosthesis	procsthesis	procthesis
2. debredment	debredment	debridment	debridement
3. petechiae	pethechiae	petichiae	pettechiae
4. morphphology	morphology	morfology	morfphology
5. roncho	ronchi	rhonchi	rhoncchi
6. tonsilitis	tonsellitis	tonsillitis	tonsleitis
7. anthropometric	antropometric	anthrowpometric	amthropometric
8. luekocytes	lyekacytes	leukacytes	leukocytes
9. exkoriashun	ekoriation	excoreation	excoriation
10. aglutination	agglutination	aglutenation	aglutation

In which medical report may these statements be found?

1. Hospitalized for epididymitis 10 years ago.
2. Bleeders were clamped and electrocoagulated as they were encountered.
3. Fairly exuberant callus formation is noted laterally along the femoral shaft.

4. No evidence for significant displacement at the femoral neck.

5. DIAGNOSIS: Gallbladder, hemorrhagic chronic cholecystitis with cholelithiasis.

6. I have been asked to see a five-year-old Caucasian male who appears in mild distress due to upper extremity burn after falling into hot coals in his back yard.

7. She will be seen by Dr. Moore, who will follow her SLE and ITP.

8. Penrose drains were placed on each side of the vesical gutter.

Translate medical abbreviations using a medical dictionary or appendix.

1. not equal to ____________________

2. ♀ ____________________

3. one half ____________________

4. ♂ ____________________

5. central nervous system ____________________

6. biopsy ____________________

7. diagnosis ____________________

8. # ____________________

9. coronary artery disease ____________________

10. ℞ ____________________

Chapter 15

Additional Writing Applications

Objectives

Upon completion of this chapter, the student should be able to:

- consult various resources to do medical research
- understand the formats for writing a manuscript and grant proposal
- recognize the distinctions among writing medical ads, promotions, and announcements
- write information sheets and materials for patient information
- spell various medical terms
- translate various medical abbreviations and symbols

The diversity of writings in the medical profession is vast, ranging from a single one-page information sheet to a research paper containing multiple pages. The most common types of medical writings are:

> *Journal article:* writing on a specific topic that details background, methods, results, and conclusions; usually appears in a newspaper, journal, or magazine.
>
> *Manuscript:* a written or typewritten version of a book or other work submitted for publication.
>
> *Report:* a formal account of proceedings presented in detail.
>
> *Document:* an original written or printed page that furnishes evidence or information.
>
> *Abstract:* a short piece of writing that clearly summarizes larger works; covers procedures, results of studies or experiments, and conclusions.
>
> *Research paper:* an investigation into a topic to obtain facts or theories.
>
> *Grant proposal:* a request for a sum of money to research special projects.

Research

Research is necessary in all types of medical writing. Research is a diligent and systematic investigation into a topic to discover facts and theories. Change occurs rapidly in the development of diseases, health conditions, treatments, and technologies. Continuous research is an integral process to the advancement of medical discoveries. One- or two-year-old data are considered outdated. Some resources available are:

- Medical libraries
- Internet
- Medical periodicals
- Public health department
- Healthcare organizations
- Hospitals and clinics
- Interviews with medical personnel
- Computer technology
- Clinical studies

When researching medical literature, focus on finding the answers to these analytical questions:

What is the objective of the study?

Was the hypothesis tested?

Were convincing factors used to justify the study?

Were laboratory tests used?

What were the significant results?

Did the conclusions match the results?

What new questions resulted?

Manuscripts

Medical professionals may not be required to write original materials. However, they are routinely responsible for the mechanics, editing, and organization of multiple pages of data.

General Format Guidelines

Undoubtedly, the most challenging piece of writing to organize is the manuscript. The manuscript is a document intended for publication, either as an article in a periodical, a chapter in a book, or a complete book. When publication is under consideration, the publisher usually provides format guidelines. The main parts of a manuscript are:

Title Page	Title
	Number of authors
	For whom the manuscript is written
	Name of the affiliation, department
	Date of submission
Abstract	Brief summary of the article (100–150 words)
Introduction	Specific problem under study
	Background to clarify topic
	Rationale and purpose of the manuscript

Methods	How the study was conducted Procedure
Results	Tables and figures Statistics
Discussion	Evaluation and interpretation of results
Other Experiments	Integration of results
References	Supportive interpretations cited
Appendix	Supplementary information

APA Writing Style

Manuscripts written about topics in the medical field should follow the American Psychological Association (APA) style of writing. Anyone writing a manuscript should secure a copy of the *Publication Manual of the American Psychological Association.*

A copy can be obtained from:

American Psychological Association
Book Order Department
P.O. Box 92984
Washington, DC 20090-2984

Telephone 800.374.2721 FAX 202.336.5502

Web site:

www.apa.org/books/ordering

Consider these basic APA guidelines when organizing and editing a manuscript:

- Standard white bond paper, 8½ by 11 inches,
- One inch margins on top, bottom, left and right sides
- Lines typed unjustified, or uneven (ragged) at the right margin
- Pages numbered consecutively in upper right-hand corner, using Arabic numerals.
- Pages arranged in the following order:
  Title page (page 1)
  Abstract is on a separate page (number 2)
  Text starts a new page, beginning on page 3
  References

Title Page

On the title page, the main title is typed in uppercase and lowercase letters. If the main title is more than one line, use a double space between the lines. An abbreviated version of the title is called a running head, which may be used for identification of the article on subsequent pages. The name of the author appears on a separate line. If the author of the manuscript is not affiliated with an institution, the city and state of the author is used instead.

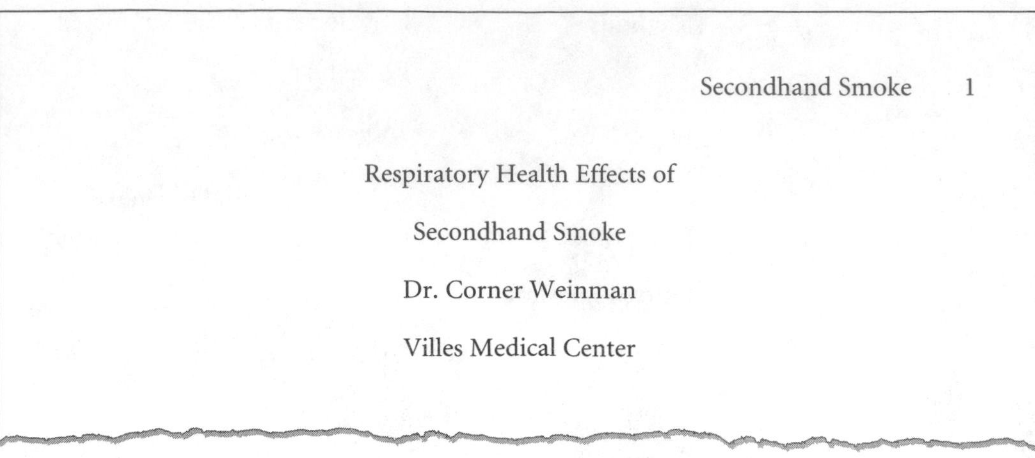
Secondhand Smoke 1

Respiratory Health Effects of

Secondhand Smoke

Dr. Corner Weinman

Villes Medical Center

Figure 15-1 Manuscript Title Page

Abstract Page

The word "abstract" is centered on the abstract page (Figure 15-2). A running head is used, and the text is one paragraph in block form, double-spaced.

Text Page

On the first page of text (Figure 15-3), the title is centered, one double space below the short title. The first line of the text is one double space below the main title.

Reference Page

A reference list is a list (Figure 15-4), of all sources cited in a manuscript. (In contrast, a bibliography lists further readings or other works not specifically cited in the text.) References are placed in alphabetical order by the author's last name. The first names are abbreviated. The first line of an item is indented and subsequent lines are flush with the left margin. All typing is double space.

Citations

When facts, opinions, and ideas of others are referred to in a manuscript, it is necessary to acknowledge the source. If a writer quotes or paraphrases a fact or idea in a text, the author's last name, the year of publication, and, if applicable, a page number are cited parenthetically.

Secondhand Smoke 2

Abstract

The overall percentage of people affected by secondary smoke has reached alarming proportions according to this study . . .

Figure 15-2 Manuscript Abstract Page

Secondhand Smoke 3

Respiratory Health Effects of

Secondary Smoke

The first recorded use of tobacco appeared over a thousand years ago on Mayan stone carvings. History also records that Columbus saw natives roll, light, and smoke tobacco . . .

Figure 15-3 First Page of Text of Manuscript

Secondhand Smoke 30

References

McGinnis, J. M. (1997). Health progress in the United States. *Journal of the American Medical Association, 46* (4), 130–132.

Lo, B. (2000). Behind closed doors: promises and pitfalls of ethics committee, *New England Journal of Medicine, 28* (2), 150–167.

Figure 15-4 First Page of Reference List of Manuscript

Examples

"Furthermore, Parker (1988) found that. . ."

"Diseases have been reported to increase (Momfort, 1989)."

"In a study conducted in this city, Wahlen and Pyne (2000) found that. . ."

Dr. Villes determined that the cause was due to "inadequate diet" (Smith), 1997, p. 189.

The *Publication Manual of the American Psychological Association* covers text reference citations and reference lists in great detail.

Grant Writing

Health facilities, like most other community service organizations, seek funding from private foundations and corporations, or from government programs for various projects or specific medical research endeavors. Funding source requirements differ in length and format. However, the same types of information are generally required. A simple, basic format and logical approach to planning and writing a grant is explained in this chapter.

Further information about grants may be obtained form:

www.tgci.com/publications/puborder

www.synapseadaptive.com

www.techwriteinc.com

www.revisions-grants.com

A simple format to follow when writing a grant is:

1. Proposal Summary
2. Introduction
3. Problem Statement
4. Goals and Objectives
5. Methods
6. Evaluation
7. Future Funding
8. Budget
9. Appendix

Proposal Summary

The "Proposal Summary" briefly summarizes the whole proposal text. It is the first thing a grant reviewer reads, either in the few opening paragraphs of a letter or as a larger section within a more formal proposal. The summary provides the first impression, so it should be good.

Introduction

The introductory component reinforces the connection between the requesting organization and the granting organization. The requesting organization uses this section to build its credibility, which may be more important than the rest of the proposal. Points to include:

- History of the organization
- Uniqueness of the agency
- Significant accomplishments
- Scope of financial support
- Successful related projects
- Support received from other individuals and organizations

Problem Statement

The section stating the problem deals with specific societal issues outside the organization that could be addressed if funds were granted (issues of homelessness, children with AIDS, violence among youth). Make sure the problem is realistic, and that it can be achieved in reasonable time with reasonable funds. Demonstrate knowledge of the problem with data and quotes from experts nationally and locally.

Goals and Objectives

Goals are general statements that offer the reader a broad picture of the problematic issue. Because goals are broad, they cannot be measured as stated.

Examples

Reduce teenage smoking.

Enhance reading skills of children with learning disability.

Objectives are specific, measurable outcomes of the program; the promises made to improve the conditions in the problem statement.

Examples

Reduce teenage smoking by 20%.

Within one year, children with learning disabilities will increase their reading ability by two grade levels.

The specifics of the objectives should realistically estimate the amount of benefit expected from a program. One way to define specific objectives is to project where the agency could be a year or two in the future.

Methods

"Methods" explains what strategies need to be implemented to bring about the desired results. This section gives the reader a picture of exactly how things will work and look. Justify the methodology by stating why certain strategies were chosen over others.

Evaluation

An evaluation serves two purposes. The first is that it measures the results of the proposal. The second is that it can also provide information to make changes or adjustments in the program as it moves along. To do this, the evaluation plan is implemented at the time the program starts.

Having an outside organization perform the evaluation is an option. An outside evaluation gives a more objective viewpoint and adds more credibility to the proposal.

Future Funding

The "Future Funding" component explains what happens to the program after the grant money is spent, unless it is a one-time only request. Present a plan that assures there is life after the grant is completed.

Budget

A budget is a list of expenditures during a given period. Funds to run a program fall into three categories:

1. Personnel: salaries and wages for full or part-time staff, including fringe benefits, consultants, and contract fees. These expenses may be determined by comparing salaries

to similar services elsewhere. In-kind services should be listed; that is, matching support contributions by the requesting agency.

2. Nonpersonal expenses: rent for space, lease or purchase of equipment, travel, hotel, meals, printing, and professional association membership or dues.
3. Indirect costs: costs not readily identifiable but necessary to the operation of the whole fall into this category; for example, phone costs and general supplies.

Appendix

An appendix is a collection of supplementary materials provided at the end of the proposal. (Refer to the appendixes at the end of this book as examples.) Grantors may stipulate what to include in this section, such as:

Financial audit	List of board of directors
Nonprofit status	Organizational plan
Timelines	Letters of support, endorsement
Resumes	Job descriptions

❁ ❁ ❁

Many agencies that rely on grants for support often contract the services of a professional grant proposal writer. Otherwise, proposals are written by the personnel of the requesting organization. The role of medical assistants, however, is to organize information given to them into an acceptable grant format. See Figure 15-5 for a sample grant proposal.

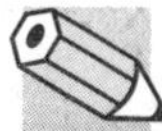

Practice 15-1

Write a short grant proposal using the format presented in the chapter.

Promotional Writing

In addition to the more structured types of writing contained in reports, research papers, grant proposals, and manuscripts, medical-related writing includes promotional types such as advertisements, press releases, announcements, brochures, and informational materials.

These items are a public or formal notice to announce a product, attend an event, give information to the public, call attention to something special, or offer goods or services. There are no limits to advertising, providing the information is true and not misleading.

Medical facilities publish promotional items in brochures, newspapers, medical journals, and publications. Data included in those items may cover:

- Philosophy
- Description of office practice
- Laboratory services
- Policy on appointments and cancellations
- Medical associations
- Policy of prescription renewal
- Map on how to get to the facility
- Park facilities

Proposal Summary

The purpose of this one-time grant is to seek $8,000 from the Davis Foundation to present a Teen Smoke-Out Program at Barry High School, in collaboration with the Villes Medical Center. The general goal of the program is to reduce smoking among students by at least 20% (30 students). The methodologies used to achieve this goal are to sponsor four two-hour seminars by a physician; to disseminate educational materials among students; to conduct a peer support group twice a month; and to offer individual counseling sessions as needed. Evaluation procedures are conducted to determine the effectiveness of the program in order to integrate it into the school's core curriculum in subsequent years.

Introduction

Nicotine is the most addictive drug used by teenagers today. Two facilities, the Villes Medical Center and Barry High School are collaborating to address this issue.

The Villes Medical Center, established over 25 years ago, provides a variety of medical services within the state and beyond. The Center is especially successful in providing smoking-cessation programs within educational settings. More than 87 elementary and high schools have benefited from the expertise of their qualified staff. Grants, service fees, and private donations support the center.

Barry High School is a public facility offering college, business, and technology courses to prepare students for life and work. Enrollment is approximately 500 students, with a student–teacher ratio of 1 to 15. The philosophy of the school is the total development of the student in body, mind, and spirit; that each may reach his or her full human potential.

Problem Statement

Smoking is the most serious health risk among teens today. More than 3,000 teens become smokers daily. In a given year, teens smoked 28 million cigarettes. More than 5 million teens will prematurely die because they chose to smoke. Teens who smoke are more likely to use alcohol, marijuana, and cocaine.

According to a recent health survey given at Barry High School, three out of ten students smoke—150 out of a total of 500 students. Barry High School, in collaboration with the Villes Medical Center decided to do something to reduce smoking among teens. The request of $8,000 in grant funds from the Davis Foundation is for that purpose.

Goals and Objectives

The goals of the grant are to:

1. Educate the student population on the effects of smoking.
2. Reduce the smoking rate of teens at Barry High School.

Figure 15-5 Sample Grant Proposal

The goals are to be achieved through these objectives:

1. Provide four two-hour educational Teen Smoke-out Seminars.
2. Reduce the number of teenage smokers by 20% in one year.
3. Provide an incentive to entice students to quit smoking.
4. Inform parents and elicit their support through the home.

Methods

Strategies of the program consist of:

1. Four seminars on smoking will be given by a physician from the Villes Medical Center to freshman, sophomore, junior, and senior classes during their respective assembly periods. Topics are the health effects of smoking, reasons for teen smoking, societal and individual costs of smoking, and smoking prevention. Seminars will occur in October, December, February, and April.
2. Establish a bimonthly support group facilitated by a Barry High School counselor and the Villes Medical Center smoking cessation counselor.
3. Give two additional credits in health science to smokers who committed themselves to the group process.
4. Offer individual counseling to group members as needed.
5. Provide program information to parents and ask for their support.

Evaluation

The program will be evaluated in three ways:

1. Give the health survey again to determine the number of students who quit smoking.
2. Have students fill out an evaluation sheet after each seminar.
3. Ask for continuous feedback from the bimonthly support group.

Future Funding

This grant is for one year. Seminars will be videotaped and integrated into the core curriculum in subsequent years.

Budget

Educational Materials	
Videos/Movies	$1,500
Text: Tobacco Biology and Politics by Stanton A. Glantz, Ph.D.	2,500
Pamphlets, Brochures, Charts, Modules, Information Sheets	600

Figure 15-5 Continued

Personnel		
Physician		1,200
Group Counselor		1,000
Individual Counselor		1,000
Travel		200
	TOTAL	$8, 000
In-kind Contributions		
Program Coordinator		2,000
Barry High School Counselor		1,000
Facility Space, Maintenance		700
Secretarial Services		300
	TOTAL	$4,000

Appendix

Copy of Seminar Evaluation Sheet
Resumes of Participating Personnel
Brochures: Villes Medical Center; Barry High School; May I Introduce Myself? I Am a Cigarette

Figure 15-5 Continued

- Financial policies
- Photo or logo of the facility
- Names of key medical and administrative staff
- Information to patients prior to their first visit
- Emergency room procedures
- Answering service
- Areas of specialization

Figure 15-6 is a sample advertisement and Figure 15-7 is a sample brochure. A brochure is a small pamphlet. The brochure shown as Figure 15-7 is the one used by the Villes Medical Center and Barry High School to announce the Teen Smoke-Out Seminars, *May I Introduce Myself? I Am A Cigarette.* And the following is an example of a news, or press, release:

> The Davis Foundation announced an $8,000 grant award to Villes Medical Center and Barry High School to run a series of four Teen Smoke-Out Seminars. According to a recent health survey given at Barry, three in ten teens smoke. The goal of the program during the coming year is to reduce smoking by 20%, according to Dr. Mary Louise Norman, Director of Villes Medical Center, and Emily Prior, Ph.D., school principal.

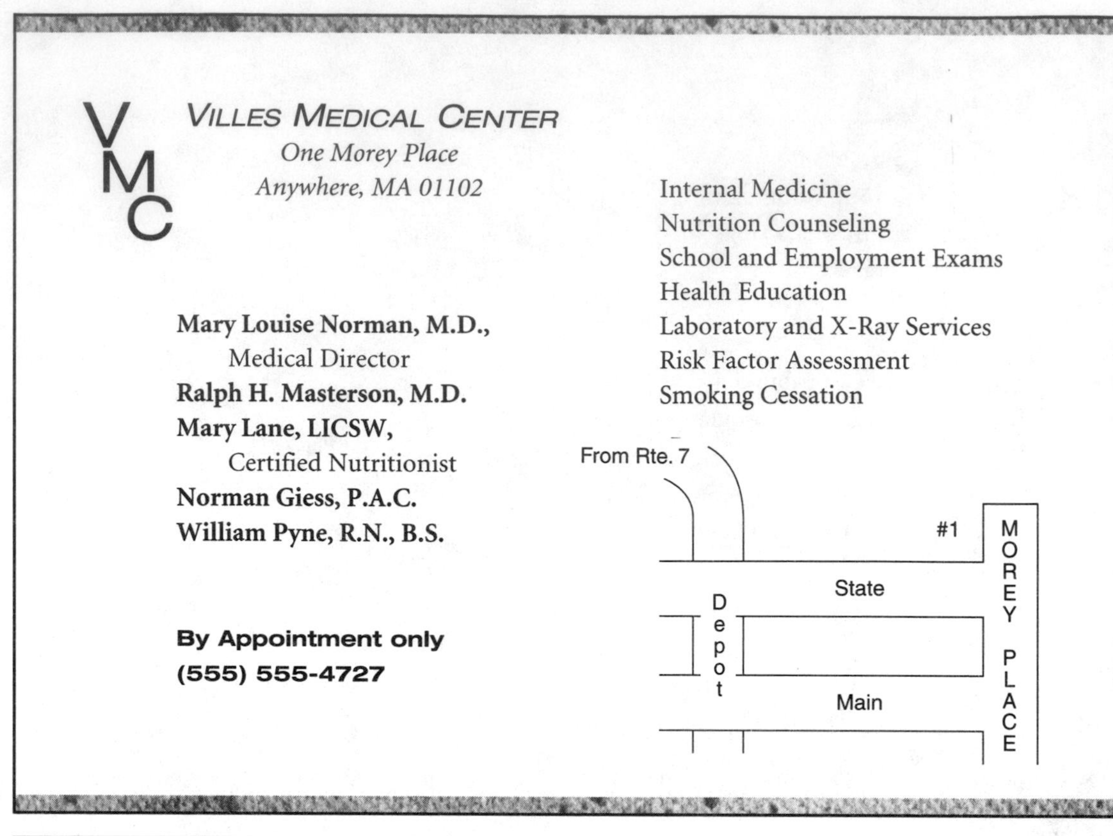

Figure 15-6 Sample Advertisement

Information sheets are a convenient way to distribute data relating to health issues. A simple format includes:

- Introduction
- Broad Topic/Narrow Topic
- Points Developed/Subtopics
- Body
- Paragraph 1
    - Topic
    - Support
    - Conclusion
    - Transitional Sentence
    - (The same format is used for additional paragraphs.)
- Conclusion
- Summary
- Ending Sentence

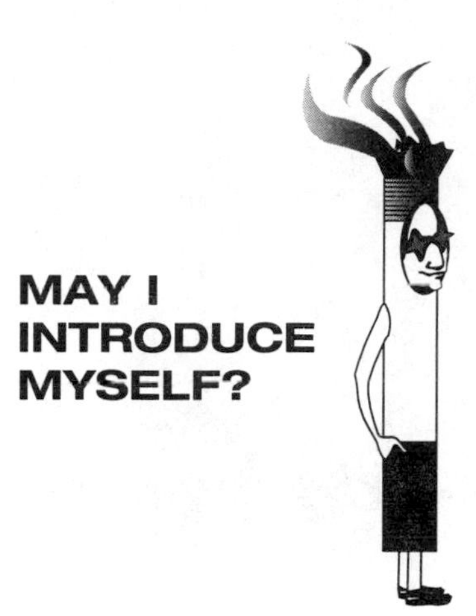

TEEN SMOKE-OUT SEMINARS
October 4, 20XX
January 18, 20XX
March 11, 20XX
May 13, 20XX

A COLLABORATION
Between
VILLES MEDICAL CENTER
and
BARRY HIGH SCHOOL

SPONSORED BY A GRANT
from the
DAVIS FOUNDATION

I AM A CIGARETTE!!

I come in many sizes and shapes, wrapped in shiny, colorful packages that are hard to resist. Advertising agencies show the public how beautiful I am, how "real cool" it is to smoke me, and how wonderful it is to be my friend. Their words flatter me:

Fashionable!

Your basic truth!

You got what it takes!

Enjoy the best of life!

You've come a long way, Baby!

Be the one with STYLE!

You can do it!

Easygoing!

Sleek!

I'm very popular. People in every walk of life respect and hold me in high esteem:

- I go to the best of parties.
- I'm the first thing people reach for in the morning and the last thing before going to bed.
- My friends even leave their homes in the middle of the night to find and smoke me. Spouses and children don't get that much attention.

Others look for me in trash cans or on the street so they can have just one more puff. So what if they get a little dirty. I'm worth it!

I'm also good. The large tobacco corporations that make me provide jobs for thousands of people. From the money you spend, I contribute millions and millions of tax dollars to the world economy. You don't feel that cost when you buy me one pack or one carton at a time. So what if over a 25-year friendship, I cost you the price of a few cars or a college degree. Friends don't let money come between them.

Like everybody else, I'm not perfect. I occasionally burn holes in clothes, rugs, and furniture, causing small fires and injuries.

What really excites me, however, are the homes I burn. The flames make such a pretty sight! Some of these fires claim the lives of my friends, but I don't worry. I'm an arsonist who can't be arrested.

I also cause bad breath, yellow teeth, hacking cough, shortness of breath, heart disease, high medical bills, and even cancer. You could die by associating with me. But don't worry, these things only happen to other people. If you should die, however, your children will give me the pleasure of their friendship by following in your footsteps.

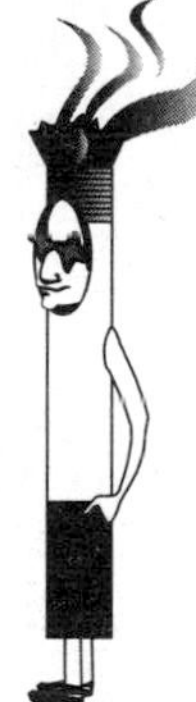

Figure 15-7 Sample Brochure

Figure 15-8 is a sample information sheet used as a handout at the Teen Smoke-Out seminars previously referred to. Its format components have been broken down and labeled for instructive purposes.

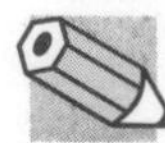

Practice 15-2

Using the format presented in the chapter, write an information sheet on any topic suggested by the instructor.

Introduction	Smoking is one of the most overpracticed addictions in the world. Most people who smoke admit that it severely injures their health, but they cannot always explain how. This information sheet briefly relates some reasons why smoking is harmful and why it should be stopped at all costs.
Broad topic:	Smoking
Narrow topic:	Dangers of not smoking; benefits of not smoking
Points developed:	Contents of a cigarette; how a cigarette works in the body; rewards of not smoking
	Body, Paragraph 1
Topic **Support**	Tobacco wrapped in paper for the purpose of smoking is a lethal weapon. A cigarette is made up of thousands of different chemicals including ammonia (cleaning fluid), nicotine (insecticide), formaldehyde (embalming fluid), arsenic (poison), carbon monoxide (car exhaust), and methanol (wood alcohol). Why do people smoke when they know these chemicals are harmful?
Transition	Consider how nicotine works in the body.
	Paragraph 2
Topic **Support**	Nicotine hits the brain and makes the smoker feel relaxed and pleasant. The inhaled smoke carries nicotine into the lungs. The blood in the lungs carries the nicotine into the heart and brain—all within seven seconds! Nicotine passes quickly and easily through the entire body in three days. It leaves the bloodstream through the kidneys. If nicotine from ten cigarettes gets trapped in the bloodstream, it would be strong enough to kill a person.
Conclusion	Each year, smoking kills more people than AIDS, alcohol, drug abuse, car crashes, murder, suicide, and fire combined.
Transition	Consequently, people have much to gain by not smoking.
	Paragraph 3
	When people quit smoking, their energy improves, they breathe better, the heart works easier, pulse rate and blood pressure become lower, and body circulation improves. The risk of heart attacks and cancer lesson by 90%. More oxygen goes to the brain and the rest of the body, and one's sense of taste and smell improves.
Conclusion	In other words, the person gets a second chance at a quality life.
Summary	Cigarettes contain harmful chemicals that cause harm to the body, even though those chemicals make a person feel "high." More people die from smoke-related illnesses than alcohol, drugs, murder and suicide combined. After quitting, the risk of a heart attack and cancer is reduced by 90%, thus providing former smokers with a new lease on life.

Figure 15-8 Information Sheet Example

Patient Education

Numerous medical procedures are given verbally to different patients over and over again. If patients are nervous, the information is easily forgotten. To save time, reduce the number of office calls, and keep patients informed, different types of printed information are distributed. Some of the topics might include:

- Preparation for tests
- Pre- and postoperative instructions
- Diets
- How to take an enema
- Care for a wound
- How to take medications
- Side effects of medications

Health organizations across the country have free literature available to patients on request. Among these organizations are the Centers for Disease Control and Prevention, American Cancer Society, American Red Cross, American Medical Association, and the U.S. Department of Health and Human Services. Booklets, pamphlets, brochures, and magazines are also disseminated through physicians' offices or other health-care facilities. Figure 15-9 is a sample pamphlet about cholesterol.

Medical Spelling

Become familiar with the spelling of the following words:

abrasion
abscess
alkalosis
antidote
anuria
crepitation
ecchymosis
emphysema
endogenous
exogenous
familial
fibrillation
glucagon
hematoma
hematuria
hemoptysis
hereditary
inoculate
insidious
integral
intrinsic
invasive
irrigation
jejunostomy
lesion
lordosis
microorganisms
micturition
noninvasive
ossification
parenteral
permeability
quadrant
requisition

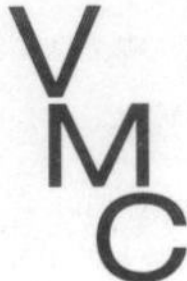

VILLES MEDICAL CENTER
One Morey Place
Anywhere, MA 01102
(555) 555-4727 Phone
(555) 555-4000 Fax

Facts About High Blood Cholesterol

High blood cholesterol is one of three controllable factors of heart disease. The other two are smoking and high blood pressure.

BECAUSE HIGH CHOLESTEROL IS CONTROLLABLE,
SOMETHING CAN BE DONE ABOUT IT.

What is cholesterol?

Cholesterol is an odorless, fatlike substance the body uses to make cell walls and hormones. The amount of cholesterol in the blood depends on two factors:

1. The amount the body produces.
2. The amount eaten in food that contains saturated fats and cholesterol.
   Saturated fats raise cholesterol. Polyunsaturated fat lowers cholesterol.

What is the danger of cholesterol?

When there is an overabundance of cholesterol in the blood, it clogs artery walls. The opening narrows. Over a period of time the heart can't get enough blood.

What is too much cholesterol?

Acceptable	less than 200
Of concern	200–239
High risk	240 and over

When cholesterol is checked, it is done on two levels: LDL and HDL. LDL (low-density lipoproteins) carries blood used in body tissues. The cholesterol in LDL is what clogs artery walls. Because of this, it is called the bad type. HDL (high-density lipoproteins) removes cholesterol from the body, preventing build up on artery walls. Because of this, HDL is called the good type.

Acceptable LDL	less than 130
Of concern	130–159
High risk	160 and over

A low HDL is a risk factor for a heart attack. The lower the HDL factors, the greater the risk.
How is cholesterol controlled?

1. Diet: eat food low in saturated fat and cholesterol. See the accompanying diet.
2. Keep weight to a good level.
3. Take prescribed medication from a physician when the diet fails.
4. Exercise regularly: a minimum of 20 minutes per day, three times a week to get results.
5. Manage stress.
6. Quite smoking.
7. Have cholesterol checked regularly.

Figure 15-9 Sample Patient-Education Pamphlet

Low Fat Diet

Food	***Acceptable***	***Unacceptable***
Beverages	Fat free buttermilk, carbonated drinks, cereal beverage, tea, coffee, skim milk	Whole milk
Bread	Any, saltines, soda crackers	Breads with eggs and large amounts of fat
Cereal	Most	None
Dessert	Angel-food cake, gelatins, ices, sherbet made with skim milk	Chocolate, cocoa desserts
Fat	Salad dressing and oil, tub margarine	Cream, butter
Fruit	Most	Avocado
Meat, fish	Lean beef, chicken, lamb, turkey, veal, fish, shellfish	Fat or fried meat, fish, or fowl, fish canned in oil
Eggs, cheese	Dry cottage, egg whites	All other cheeses, egg yolks
Potato	Most	Egg noodles, potato chips, fried potato
Soups	Clear, fat-free broth, soup made with skim milk	Those containing cream, fat, or whole milk
Sweets	Candy, jam, jelly, marmalade, molasses, syrups, sugar	Those made with cream, chocolate, cocoa, fat, nuts
Vegetables	Any	None
Other	Catsup, chili sauce, pickles, popcorn (unbuttered) vinegar, spices	Gravy, nuts, olives, white sauce, peanut butter

Figure 15-9 Continued

resection	vascular
scoliosis	void
synovial	wound

Additional Writing Applications Study Summary

Research	**Resources:**
Investigation into a topic to discover facts and theories.	Medical libraries, the Internet, medical periodicals, public health departments, healthcare organizations, hospital and clinics, interviews with medical personnel, computer technology software, and clinical studies.
Promotional Writing	**Promotional items:**
Formal notice to announce a product or event, provides information, call attention to, or offer goods or services.	Brochures, newspapers, medical journals, and publications, advertisements, news releases, and information sheets.
Patient Education	**Sample topics:**
Printed information used to inform patients about different medical topics.	Preparation for tests, pre- and post operative instructions, diets, how to take an enema, care for a wound, how to take medications, and the side effects of medications.

General Manuscript Components

Title Page	Title, author(s), affiliations, submission date, for whom written
Abstract	100–150 word summary
Introduction	Problem under study, background, purpose, rationale
Methods	How the study was conducted, procedure
Results	Tables and figures, statistics
Discussion	Evaluation and interpretation of results
Other experiments	Integration of results
References	Supportive interpretations
Appendix	Supplementary materials

Grant Proposal Components

Proposal Summary	A proposal abstract briefly describing the organization seeking funds, the scope of the project, and the cost
Introduction	Background of the applicant organization, scope of financial support, related projects, and other support received
Problem Statement	Situation or problem to be solved through the proposed grant; the cause for which the proposal was written

Goals and Objectives	Goals: broad and unmeasurable statements that give a general focus to the grant program Objectives: specific and measurable outcomes of the situation
Methods	Detailed activities that will take place in order to achieve the objectives of the program
Evaluation	Tools to determine how effective the program was in reaching its goals.
Future Funding	How the program will continue when the money runs out.
Budget	Itemized list of costs, based on the goals and objectives and strategies to implement them.
Appendix	Supplementary materials requested by the grantor

Skills Review

1. Arrange these components as they would appear in a manuscript:

   Method

   Appendix

   Abstract

   Results

   Title page

   Introduction

2. List four types of resources used in medical research:

   ______________________ ______________________

   ______________________ ______________________

3. List four types of medical writings:

   ______________________ ______________________

   ______________________ ______________________

4. Fill in each blank with the correct word from the list.

abstract	clinical study	method	grant	appendix
goal	research	manuscript	objective	citation

   A. Document intended for publication ______________

   B. Measurable outcomes from a program ______________

C. Ideas of others referred to in a manuscript ___________________

D. Sources cited in a manuscript ___________________

E. Reports about new treatment on patients ___________________

F. Strategies to bring about a result ___________________

G. A request for money to fund a special project ___________________

H. Systematic investigation into a topic ___________________

I. Collection of supplementary materials ___________________

5. Prepare either an ad, brochure, promotion, or announcement.

Circle the correctly spelled word in each line:

1.	perenteral	parenteral	parenterel	peranteral
2.	microrganism	micraorganism	mikroorganism	microorganism
3.	hemaptysis	hemoptysis	hemoptisis	hemaptitis
4.	micturition	mictaration	mictiration	mictoration
5.	eccymosos	echymosos	ecchymosis	ecchimosis
6.	insedious	incsidious	insidious	insideous
7.	resection	resektion	risiction	resecsion
8.	eksogenous	exoginous	exaugenous	exogenous
9.	scoleosis	scolliois	scoliosis	scoliocis
10.	reguisiton	requisition	recquisition	requisiton

Translate medical abbreviations using a medical dictionary or appendix.

1. tertiary ___________________

2. arterial blood gas ___________________

3. blood, urea, nitrogen ___________________

4. female ___________________

5. pupils equal, round, reactive to light and accommodation ____________________

6. ratios ____________________

7. secondary ____________________

8. with ____________________

9. increase ____________________

10. number ____________________

Appendix A

Spelling Rules

Spelling correctly is a real challenge. Many medical terms are long, uncommon, and somewhat tricky: *tourniquet, pneumonia, scirrhous, diarrhea, ecchymosis,* and *herniorrhaphy*. The allied health professional must be careful about spelling, especially since medical reports are legal documents. Sometimes the incorrect use of simple words like *their,* and *there* or *its* and *it's* are easily overlooked by the careful eye of the most conscientious proofreader. (In the word *conscientious,* does the *i* come before the *e* or the *e* before the *i*?)

When uncertain about how to spell a word, it should become a habit to look it up in the dictionary. A good idea for allied health workers is to keep an on-going list of spelling words that are most often misspelled in a small pocket notebook. Such lists of misspelled words are different from person to person, but the effort is rewarding.

Another helpful hint in building spelling efficiency is to divide words and spell them syllable by syllable. However, words are often misspelled because they are not pronounced correctly. In many words, letters are silent. One example is the word *often*. According to the dictionary, the first pronunciation of the word *often* sounds like *offen.* Spelling the word as it sounds is often incorrect.

Knowledge of a few basic spelling rules is helpful when documenting medical reports. Following are rules applicable in four basic areas that make spelling easier.

1. Using *ei* or *ie*
   - In most words, the letter *i* goes before *e: chief, view, piece, quiet, brief, hygiene, achieve, relief, grief, believe, review, friend, orient, belief,* and *died.*
   - The letter *i* goes before *e* except after the letter *c: receipt, receive, conceive, ceiling, perceive, deceive,* and *conceit.* Exceptions include *leisure, height, weird, seize, foreign, Alzheimers, neither,* and *either.*
   - The letter *i* goes before *e* after the *sh* sound: *shield, patient, proficient,* and *species.*
   - The letter *e* goes before *i* when *ei* sounds like the letter *a: weigh, weight, neighbor, their, heir, reign, veil,* and *eight.*
   - When the letters *i* and *e* are sounded separately, the spelling is easier: *sci-ence, a-li-en,* and *ex-pe-ri-ence.*
   - Change *ie* to *y* before adding *ing: die = dying, lie = lying.*
2. Doubling the Final Consonant

A student wrote about an experience that she had when trying to secure gainful employment as a medical assistant:

> I recently graduated from a medical assistant course and hopped to secure a position in a medical office. During one interview, I was given many pre-programed tests to determine if I possessed the potential to handle the job. I was quized on the many tasks required of a medical assistant Initially I reactted calmly to the test. It never occured to me that I would find

anything difficult. One of the exercises was to proofread a document written by a doctor who transfered a patient from one hospital to another. Because the physician refered the patient to another specialist, there was a lot of information. I only regreted the test took so long to complete. After two weeks, I was notiffied that someone else received the position. I wondered why.

The most predominant spelling error in this paragraph involves whether to double or not double the final consonant. The final consonant is doubled when the following criteria are met:

1. The word is one syllable: *fit.*
2. The word ends in a single consonant: fi*t.*
3. The final consonant is preceded by a vowel or the letter y: fit.
4. What is added (the suffix) begins with a vowel: *ed* or *ing*.

Under these conditions, the final consonant is doubled: *fitted.* Here are other examples:

ship + ed = shipped	run + ing = running
hot + ed = hottest	ship + ing = shipping

Exceptions to this rule involve words ending in the letter *w* (*showing*) or *x* (*boxed*), and the words *bus* and *gas*.

What happens to words of more than one syllable? Double the final consonant in words of more than one syllable under these conditions:

1. The accent must be on the last syllable: re*gret.*
2. The ending must be a single consonant: regre*t.*
3. The last letter is preceded by one vowel: regret.
4. What is added begins with a vowel: *ed* or *ing.*

When all these conditions are present, double the final consonant: *regretted.* Here are other examples:

transfer + ed = transferred	transfer + ing = transferring
occur + ed = occurred	occur + ence = occurrence
acquit + ed = acquitted	acquit + ing = acquitting

A critical point to remember about this rule is that a dictionary is necessary to be sure that the accent is on the last syllable of the word.

Another way to look at this rule is to identify when NOT to double the final consonant:

- When the accent is *not* on the last syllable: *of* fer, *offering.*
- The word does *not* end in a single consonant: co*ld, colder.*
- The last letter is *not* preceded by a *single* vowel: obt*ai*n, *obtained.*
- What is added does *not* begin with a vowel: *n*ess, goodness.

Examples

differ + ent = *different,* the accent is not on the last syllable.

cancel + ed = *canceled,* the accent is on the first syllable.

leap + ed = *leaped,* there are two vowels before the final consonant.

film + ed = *filmed,* ends in two consonants instead of one.

There are, of course, exceptions. Many words in the dictionary have two acceptable spellings.

Examples

travel + ers = *travelers* or *travellers*

counsel + or = *counselor* or *counsellor*

label + ed = *labeled* or *labelled*

program + ing = programming or programing

3. Adding Suffixes to a Final Silent *e*

What happens to the letter *e* at the end of a word when a suffix is added, particularly when the *e* is silent? Several rules help to answer that question.

1. Drop the final *e* before adding a suffix that begins with a vowel:

   state + ing = *stating*

   like + ing = *liking*

   use + ing = *using*

   Exceptions: eye + ing = *eyeing*

   dye + ing − *dyeing*

   shoe + ing = *shoeing*

2. Do not drop the final *e* if the suffix begins with a consonant:

   state + ment = *statement*

   like + ness = *likeness*

   use + ful = *useful*

   awe + some = *awesome*

   Exceptions: judge + ment = judgment

   acknowledge + ment = acknowledgment

3. Do not drop the *e* from words ending in *ce* or *ge* when adding *able* or *ous:*

   notice + able = *noticeable*

   outrage + ous = *outrageous*

4. Drop the *e* before adding the suffix *y:*

   edge + y = *edgy*

   ice + y = *icy*

5. When the word ends in *ie* and the suffix begins with *i,* change the *i* to *y* and add the suffix:

   vie + ing = vying

   untie + ing = untying

4. Adding Suffixes to Words Ending in *y* and *c*

- For words ending in *y* preceded by a consonant, change the *y* to *i* before adding a suffix:

  fancy + ful = fanc*i*ful

  glory + ous = glor*i*ous

  accompany + ment = accompan*i*ment

  happy + ness = happ*i*ness

  Exception: shy + ness = *shyness*

- For words ending in *y* preceded by a vowel, keep the *y* before adding the suffix:

  annoy + ance = annoyance

  obey + ed = obeyed

Although these four basic rules seem lengthy, common sense dictates their usage. They concretize and reinforce spelling habits writers already practice.

Appendix B

Capitalization Rules

Capitalize the following except as noted:

Rule	Example
The pronoun *I*	After *I* read the book, you can have it.
The first word in a sentence	*P*oems are made by fools like me.
The first word in any line of poetry	*B*ut only God can make a tree.
People's names	*R*oberta, *F.* *S*cott *F*itzgerald
Titles as part of a person's name	*S*enator Kennedy, *P*rime *M*inister Abouti
Do *not* capitalize a title used without a person's name.	secretary of state, the senator from Ohio
Words like mother, father, aunt, uncle used alone.	I asked *M*other to go.
Do *not* capitalize family members when accompanied by a possessive pronoun.	I asked my *m*other to go.
Title after a name	Jonathan Harlan, *M.D.*, Randy Kane, Jr.
Geographic names, streets, towns, and regions of a country.	*C*hina, *D*ade *C*ounty, *W*est *S*ide, the *S*outheast, *R*odeo *D*rive, *F*rance, *A*tlantic *O*cean
Do *not* capitalize directions.	Drive *w*est. Face *s*outh.
Languages, races.	*S*panish, *F*rench accent, *B*lack history
Do *not* capitalize *the* before these names.	*t*he Nile River, *t*he French people
Important buildings or structures	*V*ietnam *M*emorial, *T*rump *T*ower
Historical ages, events	*R*omantic *E*ra, *S*enior *P*rom
Do *not* capitalize *the* before these names.	*t*he Senior Prom
Names of products	*A*von, *B*ayer
Names of companies, stores, banks	*D*elta *A*irlines, *M*ercy *M*edical *C*enter, *P*athology *D*epartment, *F*ord truck

Names of specific courses	English Grammar 101
Do not capitalize subject matter.	English grammar.
Organizations	American Medical Association, Special Olympics
Political parties	Democrat, Republican
Religions, deity, worshipped figures	Baptist, Judaism, Catholicism, Buddha, Christ, Allah, God, Bible, Promised Land
Important words in the title of a book, movie, etc.	Bill of Rights, Gray's Anatomy
Unless they are the first word in a title, a, an, the, of, and, from, to, are not capitalized.	The Grapes of Wrath, The Return of the Native
Holidays, days of the week, months	Christmas, Sunday, July, Hanukkah
Do *not* capitalize seasons.	spring, summer, winter, fall
Do *not* capitalize academic years.	freshman, sophomore, junior, senior
First word in a direct quote	"The pain is here," said Mary. Mary said, "The pain is here."
Do *not* capitalize the first word of the continuation of an interrupted quote.	"The pain," said Mary, "*i*s in the stomach."
Eponyms	Parkinson's disease, Babinski's reflex, Apgar score, Fowler's position, Bell's palsy, Epstein-Barr virus
Certain abbreviations	B.C. Ph.D. A.D. M.D.

Appendix C

Number Use

- In general spell out numbers ten and under: one, nine, six, four.
- Use figures for numbers over ten: 16, 26, 785, 591.
- Spell out numbers used as the first word in a sentence: Six x-rays were taken.
- Spell out indefinite numbers and amounts: a few hundred dollars, a bunch of fifties.
- Be consistent with numbers in a sentence: five computers and twelve scanners; 5 computers, 16 scanners, and 24 lap tops.
- When two numbers modify the same noun, spell out one (the shorter number) and use numerals for the other: We mailed over 200 five-page reports.
- Separate unrelated numbers with a comma: On July 1, 28 people were laid off from work.
- A fraction alone is written in words with a hyphen: Three-fourths of the population go to bed hungry.
- Use numerals for mixed fractions: Give her 1½ ounces of medicine.
- Use figures with a.m., p.m: 11:30 a.m., 6:15 p.m.

  Note: Omit :00 on the hour time: 7 a.m.

  Do not use a.m. and p.m. with the word *o'clock*: The meeting is at 4 o'clock.
- Always use figures with symbols and abbreviations: pH 7.5, 33%, # 21 gauge, 2 cc. t.i.d., 3+, pulses 2+.
- Use figures with drugs: Give 75 mg of meperidine IM STAT.
- When the day precedes the month, use ordinal endings (th, rd, nd, st): The 2nd of February is my anniversary.
- Spell out an ordinal with no month: It is my twenty-eighth wedding anniversary.
- Spell out street names under 10. Fifth Avenue
- Use numerals for all house numbers but one: She lives at One 24th Street.
- Use numerals for money: 45 cents, $3.45, $15 for membership.

  Notes: Use the word *cents* for amounts under a dollar. Use a dollar sign for money over one dollar. Omit .00 with even dollars.
- Use numerals for ages: The patient is 46 yrs. old. John is 16 years and 2 months old.
- Use numerals with numbers that have decimal fractions: An incision was made 4.5 cm below. . . .

  Note: Always put a zero before a decimal that is not a whole number: Two capsules of Marcaine 0.2% were used.
- Dimensions, sizes, and temperature readings are expressed in figures: 43° below zero; My shoe size is 6½ and I weigh 120 lbs.

Arabic and Roman Numerals

1	I	20	XX
2	II	30	XXX
3	III	40	XL
4	IV	50	L
5	V	60	LX
6	VI	70	LXX
7	VII	80	LXXX
8	VIII	90	XC
9	IX	100	C
10	X	200	CC
11	XI	300	CCC
12	XII	400	CD
13	XIII	500	D
14	VIV	600	DC
15	XV	700	DCC
16	XVI	800	DCCC
17	XVII	900	CM
18	XVIII	1000	M
19	XIX		

Appendix D

Clichés

A cliché is a word or phrase that has lost its effectiveness through overuse. There are thousands of clichés in the English language. Following are some examples:

after all is said and done
as luck would have it
as old as the hills
at a later date
better late than never
busy as a bee
by leaps and bounds
calm before the storm
cart before the horse
cool as a cucumber
crystal clear, clear as a bell
days are numbered
dead as a doornail
don't rock the boat
easier said than done
few and far between
finger in every pie
fish out of water
flat as a pancake
fly off the handle
food for thought
fresh as a daisy
golden opportunity
good as my word
grin and bear it
in a nutshell
in one ear and out the other
in the final analysis
in the nick of time
it goes without saying
knowing the ropes
lap of luxury
last but not least
lesser of two evils
light as a feather
miss the boat
more than meets the eye
no time like the present
playing with fire
put your foot in your mouth
quick as a wink
raining cats and dogs
red as a beet
regular as clockwork
safe and sound
see eye to eye

short and sweet
shot in the arm
sink or swim
skating on thin ice
snug as a bug in a rug
so far so good
straight as an arrow
tough as nails
without rhyme or reason

Because clarity and conciseness are so essential in medical documentation, clichés should not be used. Notice how clichés in this memo distort its meaning:

Re: Stress Management Workshop

Believe it or not, Williams Hospital is offering a workshop on Stress Management. The cost of the workshop is a drop in the bucket compared to the benefits received. Applicants will come through with flying colors and learn how to be good to themselves. First and foremost, they will learn how to relate to difficult people, save time, and handle stress. This is just the icing on the cake. If you should feel that you are not satisfied, your costs will be returned. Leave no stone unturned. Openings are few and far between. Put your best foot forward and apply today.

Appendix E

Titles and Salutations

Effective letters require that the appropriate titles and salutations be used.

Position or Title	Styling for Address	Styling for Salutation
Executive branch of the Federal government		
The President	The Honorable (full name) President of the United States The White House	Dear Mr. President:
Wife of President	Mrs. (full name) The White House	Dear Mrs. (surname):
Vice President	The Honorable (full name) Vice President of the United States	Dear Mr. Vice President:
Cabinet member	The Honorable (full name) Secretary of ________________ The Secretary of ________________	Dear Mr. Secretary:
Attorney General	The Honorable (full name) The Attorney General	Dear Mr. Attorney General:
Postmaster General	The Honorable (full name) The Postmaster General	Dear Mr. Postmaster General:
Commissioner	The Honorable (full name) Commissioner of ________________	Dear Mr. Commissioner: Dear Madam Commissioner: Dear Mr. (full name): Dear Ms. (full name):
Chief Justice	The Honorable (full name) The Chief Justice of the United States	Dear Mr. (Madam) Chief Justice:
Federal judge	The Honorable (full name) Judge of ________________	Dear Judge (surname):
Director or head of an agency	The Honorable (full name) (title, name of agency)	Dear Mr./Mrs./Ms.
Congress		
Senator	The Honorable (full name) United States Senate	Dear Senator (surname):
Representative	The Honorable (full name) House of Representatives	Dear Representative (surname):

Position or Title	Styling for Address	Styling for Salutation
Speaker of the House	The Honorable (full name) Speaker of the House of Representatives	Dear Mr. Speaker: Dear Madam Speaker:
Chairman of a Committee	The Honorable (full name) Chairman of ________________	Dear Mr. Chairman: Dear Madam Chairman:
Librarian of Congress	The Honorable (full name) Librarian of Congress	Dear Mr./Mrs./Ms. (surname):
American diplomatic officials		
Ambassador	The Honorable (full name) American Ambassador	Dear Mr./Madam Ambassador
Minister	The Honorable (full name) American Minister	Dear Mr./Madam Minister:
Chargé d'Affaires	(full name), Esq. American Chargé d'Affaires	Dear Mr./Madam Chargé d'Affaires:
Consul	(full name), Esq. American Consul	Dear Mr./Mrs./Ms. (surname):
Representative to United Nations	The Honorable (full name) United States Representative to the United Nations	Dear Mr./Mrs./Ms. (surname):
Foreign diplomatic officials		
Foreign Ambassador	His/Her Excellency (full name)	Dear Mr./Madam Ambassador:
British Ambassador	His/Her Excellency The Right Honorable (full name)	Dear Mr./Madam Ambassador:
Chargé d'Affaires	Mr./Mrs./Ms. (full name) Chargé d'Affaires of ________________	Dear Mr./Madam Chargé d'Affaires:
Consul	The Honorable (full name) Consul of ________________	Dear Sir/Madam:
Minister	The Honorable (full name) Minister of ________________	Dear Mr./Madam Minister:
Prime Minister	His/Her Excellency (full name)	Excellency Dear Mr./Madam Prime Minister:
Premier	His/Her Excellency (full name), Premier of ________________	Excellency Dear Mr./Madam Premier:
President of a Republic	His/Her Excellency (full name)	Excellency Dear Mr./Madame President
Secretary General of the United Nations	His/Her Excellency (full name) Secretary General of the United Nations	Dear Mr./Madam Secretary General:

Position or Title	Styling for Address	Styling for Salutation
State and local officials		
Governor	The Honorable (full name) Governor of ________	Dear Governor (surname):
Lieutenant Governor	The Honorable (full name) Lieutenant Governor of ________	Dear Mr./Mrs./Ms. (surname):
Secretary of State	The Honorable (full name) Secretary of State of ________	Dear Mr./Madam Secretary:
Chief Justice of the State Supreme Court	The Honorable (full name) Chief Justice, Supreme Court of the State of ________	Dear Mr./Madam Chief Justice:
State Senator	The Honorable (full name) The Senate of ________	Dear Senator (surname):
State Representative	The Honorable (full name) House of Representatives	Dear Mr./Mrs./Ms.:
State Treasurer	The Honorable (full name) Treasurer of (state)	Dear Mr./Mrs./Ms. (surname):
Local Judge	The Honorable (full name) Judge of the Court of ________	Dear Judge (surname):
Mayor	The Honorable (full name) Mayor of ________	Dear Mayor (surname):
City Attorney	The Honorable (full name) (title) for the City of ________	Dear Mr./Mrs./Ms. (surname):
Commissioner	The Honorable (full name) Commissioner of ________	Dear Commissioner (surname):
Councilperson	The Honorable (full name) Councilman/Councilwoman	Dear Mr./Mrs./Ms. (surname):
Academic officials and professionals		
President of a university or college	President (full name)	Dear Dr. (surname):
President who is a priest	The Very Reverend (full name)	Dear Father (surname).
Chancellor of a university	Dr./Mr./Mrs./Ms. (full name)	Dear Dr./Mr./Mrs./Ms. (surname):
Dean of a school, university, or college	Dean (full name)	Dear Dean (surname):
Professor (with doctorate)	Dr. (full name) Professor of ________	Dear Dr. (surname):
Professor or instructor with no doctorate	Mr./Mrs./Ms. (full name)	Dear Mr./Mrs./Ms. (surname):

Position or Title	Styling for Address	Styling for Salutation
Attorney	Mr./Mrs./Ms. (full name) Attorney at Law	Dear Mr./Mrs./Ms. (surname):
Physician or surgeon	(full name), M.D. or Dr. (full name)	Dear Dr. (surname):
Dentist	(full name), D.D.S. or Dr. (full name)	Dear Dr. (surname):
Veterinarian	(full name), D.V.M. or Dr. (full name)	Dear Dr. (surname):
Certified public accountant	(full name), C.P.A.	Dear Mr./Mrs./Ms. (surname):
Engineer or scientist with doctorate	Dr. (full name), (title)	Dear Dr. (surname):
Members of the clergy		
Pope	His Holiness the Pope	Your Holiness:
Archbishop	The Most Reverence (full name) Archbishop of ________________	Dear Archbishop (surname):
Archdeacon	The Venerable (full name) Archdeacon of ________________	My Dear Archdeacon:
Cardinal	His Eminence Cardinal (full name)	Your Eminence:
Bishop, Roman Catholic	The Most Reverend (full name)	Dear Bishop (surname):
Bishop, Episcopal	The Right Reverend (full name)	Dear Bishop (surname):
Bishop, other denominations	The Reverend (full name) Bishop of ________________	Dear Bishop (surname):
Dean of a cathedral	The Very Reverend (full name) Dean of ________________	Dear Dean (surname):
Priest	The Reverend (full name)	Dear Father (surname):
Minister or pastor	The Reverend (full name)	Dear Reverend (surname):
Rabbi	Rabbi (full name)	Dear Rabbi (surname):
Mother Superior	The Reverend Mother Superior Convent of ________________	Reverend Mother:
Sister, Roman Catholic	Sister (full name), (order)	Dear Sister (full name):
Military chaplain	Chaplain (full name) (rank and service)	Dear Chaplain (surname):
Military ranks		
General*	General (full name) (branch of service)	Dear General (surname):

*It is common practice to show the specific rank, such as Major General; Lieutenant General; Rear Admiral; Vice Admiral; First Lieutenant; Lieutenant, j.g., if that rank is known to the sender. This distinction, however, is not made in the salutation.

Position or Title	Styling for Address	Styling for Salutation
Admiral*	Admiral (full name) (branch of service)	Dear Admiral (surname):
Colonel	Colonel (full name) (branch of service)	Dear Colonel (surname):
Major	Major (full name) (branch of service)	Dear Major (surname):
Captain	Captain (full name) (branch of service)	Dear Captain (surname):
Commander	Commander (full name) (branch of service)	Dear Commander (surname):
Lieutenant*	Lieutenant (full name) (branch of service)	Dear Lieutenant (surname):
Chief Warrant Officer	Chief Warrant Officer (full name) (branch of service)	Dear Mr./Ms. (surname):
Petty Officer	Petty Officer (full name) (branch of service)	Dear Mr./Ms. (surname):
Ensign	Ensign (full name) (branch of service)	Dear Ensign (surname):
Master Sergeant	Master Sergeant (full name) (branch of service)	Dear Sergeant (surname):
Cadet	Cadet (full name) (branch of service)	Dear Cadet (surname):
Midshipman	Midshipman (full name) (branch of service)	Dear Midshipman (surname):

*It is common practice to show the specific rank, such as Major General; Lieutenant General; Rear Admiral; Vice Admiral; First Lieutenant; Lieutenant, j.g., if that rank is known to the sender. This distinction, however, is not made in the salutation.

Appendix F

Proofreaders' Marks

Symbol	Meaning	Edited Sample	Corrected Sample
ds[	double space	ds[Cervical ROM remained pain free.	Cervical ROM remained pain free.
ss[	single space	ss[Headache disorder was due to his neck injury.	Headache disorder was due to his neck injury.
(ital)	use italic print	(ital) Journal of Medicine	*Journal of Medicine*
⊙	insert a period	Dr William Bradley	Dr. William Bradley
¶	new paragraph	. . . protein balance. ¶Rice and beans . . .	. . . protein balance. Rice and beans . . .
⁀	delete a space	en docrine	endocrine
○	spell out	(2) pills per day	two pills per day
∽	transpose	Alhzeimer	Alzheimer
∧	insert a word	program ∧ physical therapy (of)	program of physical therapy
≡	capitalize	Mary w. Jackson	Mary W. Jackson
ℓ	delete a word	~~high~~ temperature of 103	temperature of 103
/	lower case letter	allergic to Penicillin	allergic to penicillin
=	insert a hyphen	state-of-the art technology	state-of-the-art technology
—	insert underscore	issue of Time	issue of <u>Time</u>
bf ~~~	bold face print	the lymphatic (bf)	the **lymphatic** system
∧,	insert a comma	sensitive caring nurse	sensitive, caring nurse
∨'	insert an apostrophe	Hodgkins disease	Hodgkin's disease
#∧	insert space	according tothe final . . .	according to the final . . .
∧	insert a letter	body tempeture (a)	body temperature

Appendix G

Instructor's Symbols for Correction

Agreement problem	agr.
Awkward expression	awk.
Common fault	cf.
Double negative	d. neg.
Sentence fragment	frag.
Be more specific	gen.
Grammatical error	gram.
Incomplete	inc.
Not clear	n. c.
Begin paragraph	¶
Not parallel	//
Punctuation	P
Redundant	red.
Run-on sentence	RO
Sentence structure	ss
Spelling	sp.
Word choice	w. c.
Word order	w. o.
Be concise	wordy

Appendix H

Medical Abbreviations and Symbols

A thorough understanding of their meaning and proper usage is extremely important. Refer to a medical dictionary for details. Abbreviation may appear with or without periods or capital letters, depending on the facility that adopts them.

A&P	auscultation and percussion
a.c.	before meals (ante cibum)
A.D., a.d.	right ear (auris dextra)
A.S., a.s.	left ear (auris sinistra)
A.U., a.u.	both ears (aures unitas)
A	assessment
aa	of each
AAMA	American Association of Medical Assistants
AAROM	active assistive range of motion
ABD	abdomen
abd.	abduction; abdomen
ABG	arterial blood gas
ACS	American Cancer Society
ACTH	adrenocortiotropic hormone
ad lib	as desired
AD	Alzheimer's disease
ADA	American Diabetic Assocation
ADH	antidiuretic hormone
ADHD	attention-deficit hyperactivity disorder
ADL	activities of daily living
Adm	admission
AF	atrial fibrillation
AHIMA	American Health Information Management Association
AIDS	Acquired Immunodeficiency Syndrome
AIHA	autoimmune hemolytic anemia
AJ	ankle jerk
AK	above the knee
ALL	acute lymphocytic leukemia
ALS	amyotrophic lateral sclerosis (Lou Gehrig's disease)
alt. hor.	every other hour
alt. noc.	every other night
alt. dieb.	every other day
ALT	alanine amniotransferase (formerly SGPT)
AMA	American Medical Association; against medical advice

amb	ambulatory
AML	acute myelocytic leukemia
amp.	ampule
ANA	American Nurses Association, antinuclear antibody
Ant.	anterior
ap	before dinner
A-P, A&P	anterior-posterior, auscultation and percussion
aq. dest.	distilled water
AQ, aq	water
aq. frig.	cold water
AR	apical rate
ARD	atrial septal defect
AROM	active range of motion
AS	aortic stenosis
ASA	aspirin
ASAP	as soon as possible
ASCVD	arteriosclerotic cardiovascular disease
ASD	atrial septal defect
ASH, ASHD	arteriosclerotic heart disease
ASIS	anterior superior iliac spine
AST	serum aspartate amniotransferase (formerly SGOT)
A-V, AV	atrioventricular, ateriovenous
ax	axillary
B cells	lymphocytes produced in the bone marrow
b.i.d., bid	twice a day (bis in die)
b.i.n.	twice a night
B/S, BS	bedside, blood sugar, breath sounds
Ba	barium
bands	banded neutrophils
baso	basophils
BBB	bundle branch block
BE	barium enema; below the elbow
bib.	drink
bilat.	bilaterally
BK	below the knee
BM	bowel movement
BMR	basal metabolic rate
BMT	bone marrow transplant
bol.	pill
BP	blood pressure
BPH	benign prostatic hypertrophy
bpm	beats per minute
Bronch.	bronchoscopy
BRP	bathroom privileges
BT	bleeding time
BUN	blood, urea, nitrogen
Bx	biopsy
C 1 – C 7	cervical vertebrae
C	centigrade, calorie, Celsius
C&S	culture and sensitivity
C/O, co	complains of

c/w	compare with
Ca	calcium
CA	cancer; chronological age; cardiac arrest
CABG	coronary artery bypass graft
CAD	coronary artery disease
cap.	capsule
CAT scan	computed axial tomography
Cath	catheter
CBC, c.b.c.	complete blood count
CBS	chronic brain syndrome
cc	cubic centimeter
CC, C/C	chief complaint
CCU	coronary care unit
CDC	Centers for Disease Control and Prevention
CF	cystic fibrosis
cf.	compare
CHD	coronary heart disease
Chem.	chemotherapy
CHF	congestive heart failure
chol	cholesterol
chr	chronic
CIS	carcinoma in situ
CLD	chronic liver disease
CLL	chronic lymphocytic leukemia
cm	centimeter
CMA	Certified Medical Assistant
CMF	cytoxan, methotrexate, 5-fluorouracil
CNS	central nervous system
CO_2	carbon dioxide
COLD	chronic obstructive lung disease
COPD	chronic obstructive pulmonary disease
COTA	Certified Occupational Therapy Assistant
CP	cerebral palsy
CPK	creatine phosphokinase
CPR	cardiopulmonary resuscitation
CRF	chronic renal failure
C-section	cesarean section
CSF	cerebrospinal fluid
CT scan	computed tomography
CTA	clear to auscultation
CTS	carpal tunnel syndrome
CV	cardiovascular
CVA	cerebrovascular accident
CVP	central venous pressure
Cx	cervix
CX, CXR	chest x-ray
cysto	cystoscopy
5-FU	5-fluorouracil
D&C	dilation and curettage
D/C, dc	discontinue
d.	day

DD	discharge; diagnosis
DDS	Doctor of Dental Surgery
Decub	decubitus ulcer
Derm.	dermatology
DES	diethylstilbestrol
DI	diabetes insipidus
diff	differential (white blood count)
DIG	digoxin; digitalis
DM	diabetes mellitus
DMD	Doctor of Dental Medicine
DNA	deoxyribonucleic acid
DNR	do not resuscitate
DO, D.O.	Doctor of Osteopathy
DOA	dead on arrival
DOB	date of birth
DOE	dyspnea on exertion
DPT	diptheria-pertussis-tetanus vaccine
DRE	digital rectal exam
DRGs	diagnostic related groups
DTs	delirium tremens
DTR	deep tendon reflex
DUB	dysfunctional uterine bleeding
DVT	deep venous thrombosis
Dx	diagnosis
EBV	Epstein-Barr virus
ECC	endocervical curettage
ECF	extended care facility
ECG, EKG	electrocardiogram
ECHO	echocardiography
ECT	electroconvulsive therapy
EEG	electroencephalogram
EENT	eye, ear, nose, and throat
EGD	esophagogastroduodenoscopy
ELISA	enzyme-linked immunosorbant assay (AIDS test)
EM	electron microscope
EMB	endometrial biopsy
EMG	electromyogram
EMS	emergency medical service
ENT	ear, nose, throat
EOM	extraocular movement
eos., eosin	eosinophils
ER	Emergency Room
ERT	estrogen replacement therapy
ESR	erythrocyte sedimentation rate; sed rate
ESRD	end-stage renal disease
ESWL	extracorporeal shock-wave lithotripsy
ETT	exercise tolerance test
eval.	evaluation
ext.	extension
F	Fahrenheit
f	female

FACP	Fellow, American College of Physicians
FACS	Fellow, American College of Surgeons
FB	foreign body
FBS	fasting blood sugar
FDA	Food and Drug Administration
FEF	forced expiratory flow
FEV	forced expiratory volume
FHT	fetal heart tones
FHx, FH	family history
flex	flexion
FP	Family Practice
FROM	full range of motion
FSH	follicle-stimulating hormone
FU, F/U	follow-up
FUO	fever of unknown origin
FWB	full weight bearing
Fx, fx	fracture
G	gravida (number pregnancies)
g, gm	gram
GB	gallbladder
GBS	gallbladder series
GERD	gastroesophageal reflux disease
GGT	gamma-glutamyl transpeptidase
GI	gastrointestinal
gm	gram
gr	grain
Grav.1	first pregnancy
gt, gtt	drop, drops
GTT	glucose tolerance test
GU	genitourinary
guttat.	drop by drop
GYN	gynecology
H&P	history and physical
H	hydrogen
H&H	hematocrit and hemoglobin
h, hr	hour
h.s., hor. som.	hours of sleep, bedtime
H/A, HA	headache
H_2O	water
HCG	human chorionic gonadotropin
HCl	hydrochloric acid
HCT, Hct, hct	hematocrit
HCVD	hypertensive cardiovascular disease
HD	hemodialysis
HDL	high-density lipoprotein
HEENT	head, ears, eyes, nose, and throat
Hg	mercury
Hct and Hgb	hematocrit and hemoglobin
HGH, GH	human growth hormone, growth hormone (somatotropin)
HIV	human immunodeficiency virus
HOB	head of bed

hor. decub.	bedtime
HPI	history of present illness
HR	heart rate
HSV	herpes simplex virus
ht.	height
Htn., Htn	hypertension
Hx	history
I	iodine
I&D	incision and drainage
I&O	intake and output
I.U.	international unit
IBD	inflammatory bowel disease
ICSH	interstitial cell-stimulating hormone
ICU	intensive care unit
IDDM	insulin-dependent diabetes mellitus (Type I)
IHD	ischemic heart disease
IM	intramuscular
imp.	impression
inf.	infusion; inferior
INF.	interferon
INH	isoniazid
inj.	injection
instill.	instillation
IOP	intraocular pressure
IPPB	intermittent positive-pressure breathing
IQ	intelligence quotient
IT	inhalation therapy
ITP	ideopathic thrombocytopenic purpura
IUD, IUCD	intrauterine device, intrauterine contraceptive device
IV	intravenous
IVP	intravenous pyelogram
JCAHO	Joint Commission on Accreditation of Healthcare Organization
J	joule
K	potassium
kg	kilogram
KS	Kaposi's sarcoma
KUB	kidney, ureter, bladder
L, l	left; liter
L1–L5	lumbar vertebra
Lab.	laboratory
lap.	laparotomy
lb.	pound
LBP	low back pain
LDL	low-density lipoprotein
LE	lower extremity; lupus erythematosus
LFTs	liver function tests
LH	luteinizing hormone
liq.	liquid
LLL	left lower lobe
LLQ	left lower quadrant
LMP, lmp	last menstrual period

LOA	leave of absence
LOC	loss of consciousness; level of consciousness
LOM	limitation of motion
LP	lumbar puncture
LPN	Licensed Practical Nurse
LS	lumbosacral
LT	left
LTH	luteotropic hormone (prolactin)
LUL	left upper lobe
LUQ	left upper quadrant
lymphs	lymphocytes
lytes	electrolytes
m	male; meter
MA	mental age
MAO	monoamine oxidase
max.	maximal
mcg	microgram
M.D., MD	Medical Doctor
MED	minimum effective dose
meds., med.	medications
mEq	milliequivalents
mets	metastases
MFT	muscle function test
mg	milligrams
MG	myasthenia gravis
MI	myocardial infarction
min.	minimal; minute
ml	milliliter
mm	millimeter
MMR	measles, mumps, rubella
mol. wt.	molecular weight
mono	monocyte, mononucleosis
MR	medical record; mitral regurgitation
MRI	magnetic resonance imaging
MS	multiple sclerosis; mitral stenosis
MTX	methotrexate
multip	multiparous
MVR	mitral valve replacement
N	normal; nitrogen
N/V	nausea and vomiting
Na	sodium
NB	newborn
NBS	normal bowel sounds; normal breath sounds
neg	negative
neuro	neurological
nitro	nitroglycerin
NKA	no known allergies
NMR	nuclear magnetic resonance
noc	night
noct. maneq.	night and morning
non rep, n.r.	do not repeat

NPO, n.p.o.	nothing by mouth
NS	no show; normal saline
NSAID	nonsteroidal anti-inflammatory drug
NSR	normal sinus rhythm
NWB	non-weight-bearing
O&P	ova and parasites
O.D., o.d.	right eye; once daily
O.S., o.s.	left eye
O.U., o.u.	both eyes
O	objective
O_2	oxygen
OB	obstetrics
OBS	organic brain syndrome
OOB	out of bed
OP, O.P.	outpatient
OR, O.R.	operating room
ORIF	open reduction and internal fixation
Orth, Ortho	orthopedics
OT	occupational therapy; OTR (official signature for registered occupational therapist)
OTC	over the counter
oz.	ounce
P	pulse; para (number of births); phosphorus
P&A	percussion and auscultation
P.A., P/A	Physician's Assistant; posterioanterior
p.c.	after meals
P.O., po, per os	by mouth
p.r.	through the rectum
p.r.n.	whenever necessary
P	Plan
PA view	x-ray of the posteroanterior view
Palp.	palpable
Para 1,2,3	unipara, bipara, tripara
PAT	paraoxysmal atrial tachycardia
Path	Pathology
PBI	protein-bound iodine
PCP	*Pneumocystic carinii* pneumonia
PD	peritoneal dialysis
PDR	*Physicians Desk Reference*
PE, P.E.	physical examination
peds	pediatrics
per	by; through
PERRLA	pupils equal, round, reactive to light and accommodation
PFTs	pulmonary function tests
pH	hydrogen ion concentration
PHx	past history
PI	present illness; previous illness
PID	pelvic inflammatory disease
PKU	phenylketonuria
plts.	platelets
PM	post mortem; afternoon; petit mal seizures

PMN, poly	polymorphonuclear leukocytes
PND	paroxsymal nocturnal dyspnea
PNF	proprioceptive neuromuscular facilitation
PNI	peripheral nerve injury
POMR	problem-oriented medical record
pos.	positive
post.	posterior
Postop.	postoperative
PPD	purified protein derivative (test T.B.)
Preop.	preoperative
primip	primipara
pro time	prothrombin time
PROM	passive range of motion
PSA	prostate-specific antigen
PSIS	posterior superior iliac spine
PT	physical therapy
PT	pro time, prothrombin time
PTT	prothrombin time
pt.	patient
PTH	parathyroid hormone
PVC	premature ventricular contractions
PVD	peripheral vascular disease
PWB	partial weight bearing
q., q	every
q.d., qd	every day
q.h., qh	every hour
q.i.d., qid	four times a day
q.l., ql	as much as wanted
q.n., qn	every night
q.n.s., qns	quantity not sufficient
q.o.d., qod	every other day
q.p., qp	as much as desired
q.s., qs	quantity sufficient; as much as needed
q2h, q.2h.	every two hours
q3h, q.3h.	every three hours
q4h, q.4h.	every four hours
QA	quality assurance
qam.	every morning
qt	quart
quotid.	daily
R, rt., r.	right
R.A.	rheumatoid arthritis
R.N., RN	Registered Nurse
R/O, r/o	rule out
Ra	radium
RBC	red blood cell count
RD	Registered Dietician
RDS	respiratory distress syndrome
rehab	rehabilitation
REM	rapid eye movement
reps	repetitions

resp.	respiratory; respiration
Rh	Rhesus factor (blood)
RHD	rheumatic heart disease
RLL	right lower lobe
RLQ	right lower quadrant
RML	right middle lobe
RNA	ribonucleic acid
ROM	range of motion
ROS	review of systems
RQ	respiratory quotient
RROM	resistive range of motion
RT	respiratory therapist
RUL	right upper lobe
RUQ	right upper quadrant
Rx	treatment or therapy
s.o.s.	if necessary
s.q.	subcutaneous
S/P	status post, no change after
S	subjective
S-1, S-2	sacral vertebra
SA	sinoatrial
SBE	subacute bacterial endocarditis
SC, sc, s.c.	subcutaneous
sed. rt.	erythrocyte sedimentation rate
segs	segmented neutrophils
SGOT	serum glutamic oxaloacetic transaminase (See AST)
SGPT	serum glutamic pyruvic transaminase (See ALT)
SIDS	sudden infant death syndrome
sig	label the prescription
SLE	systemic lupus erythematosus
SOB	shortness of breath
sol, soln	solution
sp. gr.	specific gravity
spec.	specimen
stat, STAT	immediately
STD	sexually transmitted disease
Sx	symptoms
syr.	syrup
T	temperature
T&A	tonsillectomy and adenoidectomy
t.i.d.	three times a day
t.i.n.	three times a night
T/O, t.o., TO	telephone order
T1–T12	thoracic vertebra
tab.	tablet
TB	tuberculosis
temp.	temperature
TFT	thyroid function test
THR	total hip replacement
TIA	transient ischemic attack
tinct, tr.	tincture

TKR	total knee replacement
TLC, tlc	tender loving care; total lung capacity
TM	tympanic membrane
TMJ	temporomandibular joint syndrome
top.	topically
TPR	temperature, pulse, respiration
TSH	thyroid-stimulating hormone
TURP	transurethral resection of the prostate
Tx	treatment or therapy
UA, U/A	urinalysis
UE	upper extremity
UGI	upper gastrointestinal tract series
ung.	ointment
URI	upper respiratory infection
US, U/S	ultrasound
USP	United States Pharmacopeia
UTI	urinary tract infection
UV	ultraviolet
v	vein
V/O, VO, v.o.	verbal order
VD	venereal disease
VDRL	Venereal Disease Research Laboratory (tests)
vol.	volume
VS, V/S, v.s.	vital signs
vv	veins
w/v	weight in volume
WBC	white blood cell count
WC, w/c	wheelchair
WDWN	well-developed, well-nourished
w/d	well-developed
w/n	well-nourished
WF/BF	white female/ black female
WM/BM	white male/ black male
WNL	within normal limits
wt.	weight
x	times, multiplied by
x-match	crossmatch
YO, y/o	years old
Z	atomic number

Medical Symbols

degree	°	increased, elevated	↑
negative, deficiency	–	decreased, depressed	↓
positive, excess	+	of each	$\overline{aa}$
equal to	=	degree centigrade (Celsius)	°C
not equal to	≠	degree Fahrenheit	°F
greater than	>	infinity	∞
less than	<	take, prescription, recipe	℞
number, gauge, weight	#	plus or minus, positive or negative	±
forward	→		
backward	←		

therefore	∴
after	P
left	Ⓛ
before	$\bar{a}$
with	$\bar{c}$
without	$\bar{s}$
approximately	≈
change (or heat)	Δ
assistance (of one or of two people)	+1 +2
ratio	:
grain	gr.
tablet	tab.
one half	$\overline{ss}$
inch, second	″
feet, minute	′
reversible, back and forth	⇌ ↔
male	♂
female	♀
primary	1°
secondary	2°
tertiary	3°
divided by, per	/
parallel bars	//
right	Ⓡ

Appendix I

Use of a Thesaurus

A thesaurus is a reference book containing synonyms—words having the same or nearly the same meaning as another word—and antonyms—words meaning the opposite of another word. Words are listed alphabetically like a dictionary. The purpose of a thesaurus is to vary the expressions of the entry word in order to provide more interesting writing. The best known thesaurus is *Roget's.*

As an example, consider the entry for *medicine/medication:*

(N) Substance that helps cure, alleviate or prevent illness.

anesthetic, antibiotic, antidote, antiseptic, antitoxin, balm, biologic, capsule, cure, dose, drug, elixir, injection, inoculation, liniment, lotion, medicament, ointment, pharmaceutical, physic, pill, potion, prescription, remedy, salve, sedative, serum, tablet, tincture, tonic, vaccination, vaccine

Appendix J

Use of the English Dictionary

A dictionary is a reference or resource book that contains a great deal of information, depending on its size and organization. The most common purposes of a dictionary are to provide the definitions and correct pronunciation of words and to identify parts of speech. But a dictionary, Medical or English, may contain much more information:

- capitalization and punctuation rules (English)
- meaning of frequently used foreign terms
- history of words (etymology)
- comparisons of adjectives and adverbs (English)
- proofreaders' marks
- cross-references
- various tables and charts
- signs and symbols
- measurements
- bibliographies
- illustrations
- footnotes
- diseases (medical)
- units of measurement (medical)
- guide for writers (English)

Each word listed in the dictionary is referred to as an *entry* word, which is broken into syllables. The phonetic spelling of the word indicating its pronunciation is found in parenthesis after the entry. The part of speech is usually identified in italic print.

health (helth), *n.* condition of the body or mind with reference to soundness and vigor

To save time and facilitate the location of words in the dictionary, *guide words* are placed at the top of each page. The first guide word is the first word on the page. The second guide word is the last word on the page. All entries that fall *alphabetically* between the guide words are located on that page.

guide words: masthead __________________ maw

Unfortunately, many words are spelled incorrectly because they are spoken incorrectly. That is why the respelling of words is so important. The respelling of the word *health* shows that the letter *a* is silent. On the other hand, the respelling of the word *khaki* shows that the phonetic respelling is quite different from the entry word.

health (helth) **khaki** (kak′ē)

Note that the phonetic respelling uses symbols to assist in the pronunciation of words. To decipher the symbol, consult the pronunciation key found in every dictionary, whether at the bottom or side of each page, or in the front or back of the book. The accent mark after the first syllable (kak′) shows which syllable to stress.

The most common phonetic symbols are the long and short vowels and the *schwa* that looks like an upside down letter *e* (ə). The schwa sounds like *uh* as in the word *about* (ə bout). The vowels are *a, e, i, o, u,* and sometimes *y.* Long vowels have the sound of their own letter name. The symbol above a long vowel is a short horizontal line (¯) called a *macron.*

Examples

ā, as in *late* | ī, as in *ripe* | ū, as in *blue*

ē, as in *be* | ō, as in *note*

Short vowels have a small u-like symbol (˘) above the vowel called a *breve.*

Examples

ă, as in *bat* | ĭ, as in *it* | ŭ, as in *cut*

ĕ, as in *pet* | ŏ, as in *pot*

The symbols in the pronunciation key mean that the letters have the same sound as in vowels in these words:

ă, *pat* | oi, *boy*

ā, *pay* | ou, *cut*

âr, *car* | o͝o, *took*

ä, *father* | o͞o, *boot*

ĕ, *pet* | ŭ, *cut*

ē, *be* | ûr, *urge*

ĭ, *pit* | th, *thin, ether*

ī, *pie* | t, *attack, lateral*

îr, *pier* | hw, *which*

ō, *toe* | zh, *vision* \vi-ʒhen\

ô, *paw* | ə, *about* \ə-baut\

Appendix K

Use of the Medical Dictionary

A medical dictionary has most of the same features as an English dictionary—abbreviations, illustrations, tables, and symbols—but it focuses exclusively on medical terms and topics. Many medical entries have information beyond these features. For example, after the word *ostomy* is defined, further information is provided under subheadings titled: ostomy care, stoma care, irrigation of colostomy, and miscellaneous considerations.

Other subheadings might include nursing implications, caution, nursing diagnoses, etiology, first aid, poisoning, prognosis, systems, and treatment. An appendix further augments medical information under the titles of anatomy, phobias, nutritional value of foods, minerals and vitamins, universal precautions, physical content of elements, dietary allowances, major diagnostic category (MDC), nursing diagnosis, medical emergencies, and diagnostic-related groups.

Entry words in the medical dictionary are not divided into syllables, nor do they provide the part of speech as found in the English dictionary. However, they do have phonetic spellings. Because medical words are long and difficult to pronounce, the respelling is especially helpful.

Examples

influenza (ĭn′ floo-ĕn-ză)

physiology (fĭz″ ē-ŏl′ ō-jē)

Index